£9·47

Midwife's Pharmacopeia

Claire Banister

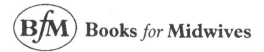

BfM Books *for* Midwives

OXFORD AUCKLAND BOSTON JOHANNESBURG MELBOURNE NEW DELHI

With thanks to the drug companies mentioned in this book
for their invaluable help in compiling this formulary

Books for Midvives
An imprint of Butterworth-Heinemann
Linacre House, Jordan Hill, Oxford OX2 8DP
225 Wildwood Avenue, Woburn, MA 01801-2041
A division of Reed Educational and Professional Publishing Ltd

ℛ A member of the Reed Elsevier plc group

First published by Books for Midwives Press 1997
Reprinted by Butterworth-Heinemann 2001

British Library Cataloguing in Publication Data
A catalogue record for this book is available from the British Library

ISBN 1 898507 61 9

Printed and Bound in Great Britain by The Cromwell Press Ltd,
Trowbridge, Wiltshire

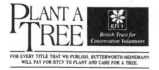

Contents

Abbreviations

b.d.	(bis die) – twice a day
t.d.s.	(ter die sumendus) – three times a day
q.d.s.	(quatre die sumendus) – four times a day
nocte	at night
stat.	immediately
p.r.n.	(pro re nata) – as the need arises
hrly	hourly
IM	intramuscular – (of injections)
IV	intravenous
IVI	intravenous infusion
p.o.	(per oram) – orally
p.r.	(per rectum) – rectally
p.v.	(per vaginum) – vaginally
s.c.	(sub cutaneous) – of injections
mg	milligrams
g	grams
kg	kilograms
ml	millilitre
CD	Controlled Drug
GSL	General Sales List
MAOI	Mono Amine Oxidase Inhibitor
NSAID	Non Steroidal Anti Inflammatory Drug
PoM	Prescription only Medicine
P	Pharmacy only Medicine
BNF	British National Formulary
DVT	Deep Vein Thrombosis
PDA	Patent Ductus Arteriosus
SLE	Systemic Lupus Erythematosus
UTI	Urinary Tract Infection
LSCS	Lower Segment Caesarean Section
ARM	Artificial Rupture of Membranes
SRM	Spontaneous Rupture of Membranes
IUD	Intrauterine Death

Drug calculations

$$\frac{\text{required strength}}{\text{available strength}} \quad X \quad \text{quantity preparation is supplied in}$$

Or

$$\frac{\text{what you want}}{\text{what you've got}} \quad X \quad \text{IT (the preparation)}$$

e.g. Ampicillin elixir 125mg/5ml
the prescription says 100mg, therefore:

$$\frac{100}{125} \quad x \quad 5 = 4\text{ml}$$

Benzl penicillin 600 mg in 5ml
the prescription says 200mg, therefore:

$$\frac{200}{600} \quad x \quad 5 = 1.66\text{ml}$$

For rates of infusion

$$\frac{\text{No. ml infused x No. drops/ml}}{\text{No. mins over which infusion is delivered}} = \frac{\text{No. drops}}{\text{delivered/min}}$$

Introduction

This book is intended for use by both midwives and student midwives. It is designed for quick reference and does not seek to replace any previously published formulary. It is therefore assumed that if a drug requires study in depth, the midwife will turn to the recognized publications, such as the British National Formulary (BNF) or the pharmaceutical companies libraries for information.

This book was written for midwives by a midwife and the preparations cited are those most frequently used in maternity units throughout the country. There is an additional page at the end of the book which can be completed with the details of drugs of specific interest or particular to the unit she works in if desired.

The chapter on miscellaneous drugs includes a very brief summary of alternative therapies but as a rule this book includes pharmaceutical preparations only.

It should also be noted that the book does not detail modes of action, uptake, ingestion, excretion etc. of preparations, although each chapter gives a brief description of the type of drug and its effects.

Drugs and the law

The legal requirements surrounding drugs and their administration should be studied separately and the midwife should become familiar with local protocols and policies for prescribing and administration. It rests with the individual midwife to become familiar with, and have working knowledge of, the preparations she works with in order to exercise her extended role of limited prescribing. This can be via Standing Orders, a list of drugs which are approved by local obstetric consultants and which the midwife can administer without the prescription by a doctor, including opioid analgesics for use in labour. There are also approved drugs which can administered by the community midwife such as antiseptics, laxatives, oxytocics and opioid antagonists.

The Midwives Rules (1993), the Midwives Code of Practice (1994) and the UKCC Guidelines for the Administration of Medicines (1992) should be adhered to when administering any drug, as should local guidelines and protocols agreed between obstetric consultants and pharmacists e.g. the administration of magnesium sulphate or ritodrine hydrochloride.

If a midwife is unfamiliar with a drug, its dosage or is concerned about the prescription e.g. the handwriting, incorrect dosage or timing, she should make her concerns known as soon as possible to the prescriber.

According to the Medicines Act (1968), the Committee on the Safety of Medicines must be satisfied that a preparation is safe and appropriate before it receives a licence. The Act governs all medicinal substances and categorizes them as follows:

1. General Sales List (GSL) – simple medicines that may be sold by any retailer.
2. Pharmacy only medicines (P) – can be sold without prescription but only by a registered pharmacist.
3. Prescription only Medicines (PoM) – these medicines can only be obtained when a prescription is issued by a medical practitioner or dentist.

Any drug which is considered addictive or which can lead to misuse is governed by the Misuse of Drugs Act 1971. This Act is concerned with the classification of controlled drugs, their possession, supply and manufacture.

Schedule 1 – hallucinogens and cannabis – these are considered without medicinal properties and are not prescribable.

Schedule 2 – morphine, cocaine, heroin and also their synthetic derivatives – prescribable but there are tight regulations on storage and prescribing and these drugs are kept on a register.

Schedule 3 – stimulants e.g. benzphetamine and also barbiturates except those used in IV anaesthesia. These require special prescription regulations except for phenobarbitone.

Schedule 4 – benzodiazepines, the group of hypnotics and anxiolytics – prescribable and do not have to be registered/kept in locked storage.

Schedule 5 – codeine and morphine combined in such small amounts with other substances that they are unlikely to cause addiction.

Controlled Drugs (CD)

These can be issued on a clients prescription chart but controls are tight. Ordering is subject to strict regulations and the drug must be accounted for at all times. Duplicates of order forms and Registers are kept for two years.

Receiving such CDs from pharmacy entails signing for and checking the amount sent and entering the new total in the Register of Controlled Drugs. Such a register is used to account for the CDs on a ward and the clients who received the drug and whether or not a drug was destroyed.

Dosage and administration must be checked and signed by two practitioners, where at least one is qualified. This means that the witness could be a student midwife.

Storage must be in a locked cupboard and preferably in a locked cupboard or locked box within that cupboard to which the keys are kept on a qualified practitioner.

The Misuse of Drugs Act 1971 and the Misuse of Drugs Regulations 1985 provide in-depth guidelines for the above outline and also make it a criminal offence to contravene the regulations. It also classifies the drugs into the harm attributable when misused.

Class A – alfentanil, cocaine, LSD, diamorphine, opium, pethidine, morphine (and any of class B which are prepared for injection).

Class B – oral amphetamines, barbiturates, cannabis resin, codeine and pholcodeine.

Class C – benzodiazepines and amphetamine related drugs.

References

British Medical Association and the Royal Pharmaceutical Society of Great Britain (1996). *British National Formulary.* No. 31, March, Avon: Bath Press.

Dimond, B. (1994). 'Medication and the midwife; statutory controls'. *Modern Midwife*, Vol. 4, No. 10, October, pp. 34–35.

Dimond, B. (1994). 'The midwifes power to prescribe'. *Modern Midwife*, Vol. 4, No. 11, November, pp. 34–35.

Dimond, B. (1994). *The Legal Aspects Of Midwifery.* Hale, Cheshire: Books for Midwives Press.

Hopkins, S.J. (1995). *Drugs And Pharmacology For Nurses*. 12th edition. Edinburgh: Churchill Livingstone.

Roch, S. (1993). 'The use of drugs by midwives'. In: Bennett, V.R., Brown, L.K. (Eds). *Myles Textbook For Midwives*. 12th edition Chapter 42, pp. 675–685. Edinburgh: Churchill Livingstone

United Kingdom Central Council (1992). *Standards For The Administration Of Medicines*. London: UKCC.

United Kingdom Central Council (1993). *Midwives Rules*. London: UKCC.

United Kingdom Central Council (1994). *The Midwives Code Of Practice*. London: UKCC.

United Kingdom Central Council (1996). *Guidelines For Professional Practice*. London: UKCC.

CHAPTER ONE

Antacids

These are drugs/preparations used to reduce gastric acidity and give relief from heartburn, when changes in diet and posture have no effect. They may also be used as prophylaxis prior to induction of anaesthesia where there is a risk of Mendelssons syndrome i.e. prior to either elective or emergency caesarean section.

H2 antagonists act upon histamine receptors and can intensify or aggravate an asthmatic response.

The student should be aware of:

- the effect of progesterone on the mother,

- local protocols for management of high risk clients during labour,

- the procedure of applying 'cricoid pressure' during induction of anaesthesia,

- updated resuscitation techniques and

- effects of narcotic analgesia on gastric emptying.

B.P.	alginic acid
Proprietary	GAVISCON ®
Group	antacid
Uses/indications	dyspepsia, cardiac reflux (heartburn)
Type of drug	GSL
Presentation	tablets, oral suspension
Dosage	tablets 1–2 as required or 10–20 ml as required
Route of admin.	oral
Contra-ind.	no data available
Side effects	no data available
Interactions	impaired absorption of oral iron
Fetal risk	nil known
Breastfeeding	not secreted in breastmilk

B.P.	cimetidine
Proprietary	DYSPAMET ®, TAGAMET ®
Group	antacid, H2 receptor antagonist
Uses/indications	to reduce gastric acidity, intrapartum or prior to CS
Type of drug	PoM
Presentation	tablets – light green, also chewable and effervescent
Dosage	*oral* – 400 mg at start of labour rptd 4 hrly (max 2.4 mg/day) *IM* – 200 mg 4–6 hrly *IV* – slow injection 200 mg over at least
Route of admin.	oral, IM, IV
Contra-ind.	avoid in clients stabilized on phenytoin and warfarin
Side effects	dizziness, rash, in high doses reversible confusional states, headache
Interactions	*analgesics* – inhibits the metabolism of opioid analgesics *anticoagulants* – inhibits the metabolism of warfarin *antiepileptics* – inhibits the metabolism of phenytoin *antihypertensives* – inhibits the metabolism of labetalol
Fetal risk	no data available
Breastfeeding	excreted in breastmilk but not known to be harmful

B.P.	ranitidine
Proprietary	ZANTAC ®, contains sodium
Group	antacid, H2 antagonist
Uses/indications	reduces gastric acidity in high risk labours
Type of drug	PoM
Presentation	tablets (also dispersible or effervescent), syrup, injection
Dosage	150 mg at onset of labour repeat 6 hrly or see protocols
Route of admin.	oral, IM, IVI
Contra-ind.	as for cimetidine, hypersensitivity
Side effects	as for cimetidine
Interactions	as for cimetidine, but effects less likely
Fetal risk	crosses the placenta and should only be used in the long term if essential, for prophylaxis in labour or LSCS. No adverse effect has been reported on labour, delivery or neonatal period
Breastfeeding	excreted in significant amounts but not known to be harmful

References

Bennett, V.R., Brown, L.K. (1993). *Myles Textbook For Midwives*. 12th edition. pp. 172, 442, 457. Edinburgh: Churchill Livingstone.

Briggs, G.G., Freeman, R.K., Yaffe, S.J. (1990). *Drugs In Pregnancy And Lactation: A Reference Guide To Fetal And Neonatal Risk*. 3rd edition. Baltimore: Williams and Wilkins.

British Medical Association and Royal Pharmaceutical Society of Great Britain (1996). *British National Formulary*. March, No. 31, Avon: Bath Press.

Enkin, M., Kierse, M., Renfrew, M., Nielson, J. (1995). *A Guide To Effective Care In Pregnancy And Childbirth*. 2nd edition. Oxford: Oxford University Press.

GLAXO ™ – data sheets – ZANTAC ® (1994)

Henney, C.R., Dow, R.J., MacConnachie, A.M. (1995). *Drugs In Nursing Practice: A-Z Guide*. Edinburgh: Churchill Livingstone.

Hopkins, S.J. (1995). *Drugs And Pharmacology For Nurses*. 12th Edition. Edinburgh: Churchill Livingstone.

Read, M.D., Golightly, P.W., Grant, E. (1996). *Drugs In Breast Milk*. 14th edition. Boehringer Ingelheim Ltd.

Further reading

Department of Health (1996). *Report On The Confidential Enquiry Into Maternal Deaths 1991–1993*. London: HMSO.

Enkin, M., Kierse, M., Renfrew, M., Nielson, J. (1995). *A Guide To Effective Care In Pregnancy And Childbirth*. Chapter 13, parts 4 and 11, Chapter 29, parts 5.2 and 7. Oxford: Oxford University Press.

Vamcr, R.G. (1993). 'Mechanisms of regurgitation and its prevention with cricoid pressure'. *International Journal Of Obstetrical Anaesthesia*, Vol. 2, No. 4, October. pp. 207–215.

CHAPTER TWO

Anaesthesia

These drugs depress part of the central nervous system, causing loss of sensation in a part of, or in the whole of, the body.

There are two main groups, inhalational and intravenous.

These drugs are a speciality of an anaesthetist, although midwives do use certain ones e.g. nitrous oxide via Entonox, or local agents such as lignocaine for perineal infiltration and bupivicaine for epidural top-ups. This chapter explores those anaesthetics used by midwives and not those administered by anaesthetists alone.

It is also of note that in the 1991–93 Department of Health Report on Confidential Enquiries into Maternal Deaths in the United Kingdom (HMSO, 1996) anaesthesia was directly responsible for eight deaths (6.2 per cent), and contributed to six (a considerable number), several of which were due to lack of careful monitoring.

Midwives need to be aware of the action of anaesthetics and units need to provide recovery areas for LSCS's patients and high-risk clients.

The student should be aware of:

*   the difference between analgesia and anaesthesia,

*   the difference between local, regional and general anaesthesia,

*   the physiology and pathophysiology of the perception of pain,

*   the physiological principles underpinning epidural anaesthesia,

*   problems occuring with obstetrical anaesthesia e.g. the effects of progesterone on the mother, the presence of two patients rather than one, the pressure of the gravid uterus,

*   updated resuscitation techniques and

*   how to apply cricoid pressure if requested to in an emergency.

B.P.	nitrous oxide
Proprietary	
Group	anaesthetic, inhalational
Uses/indications	analgesia during labour
Type of drug	PoM, standing orders
Presentation	cylinders – blue with blue and white valve end
Dosage	50% nitrous oxide, 50% oxygen, self administered via mask or Entonox equipment
Route of admin.	inhalational
Contra-ind.	nil stated
Side effects	drowsiness, nausea, vomiting
Interactions	enhances the effect of other anaesthetic or analgesic
Fetal risk	nil known
Breastfeeding	not applicable

B.P.	lignocaine hydrochloride
Proprietary	XYLOCAINE ®
Group	local anaesthetic
Uses/indications	perineal infiltration – prior to episiotomy or suturing, or for nerve blocks
Type of drug	PoM, standing orders
Presentation	ampoules, 1% or 2%
Dosage	as per unit protocol, lowest concentration and smallest dose producing the required effect
Route of admin.	injection
Contra-ind.	hypersensitivity
Side effects	hypotension, bradycardia, hypersensititvty can lead to anaphylaxis although this is rare, also inadvertant IV injection can lead to central nervous system excitory response and then drowsiness, convulsions and respiratory arrest
Interactions	*beta blockers* – increased risk of myocardial depression with propanalol *antacids* – cimetidine can impair the absorption of lignocaine into the circulation
Fetal risk	after large doses neonatal respiratory depression, hypertonia, bradycardia after paracervical block or accidental direct injection during infiltration of the perineum prior to episiotomy
Breastfeeding	not applicable

B.P.	**bupivicaine hydrochloride**
Proprietary	MARCAIN ®
Group	local anaesthetic
Uses/indications	epidural anaesthesia, spinal anaesthesia
Type of drug	PoM
Presentation	ampoules of differing percentages
Dosage	as prescribed by the anaesthetist
Route of admin.	injection
Contra-ind.	hypovolaemia, hypotension, pyogenic infection of the skin at or adjacent to the lumbar site, coagulation disorders or on going coagulation treatment
Side effects	maternal hypotension, myocardial depression and seizures if given IV? raised maternal temperature and some diminishing of uterine contractions
Interactions	*anti-arrythmics* – increased myocardial depression
Fetal risk	bradycardia, respiratory depression, fetal hypothermia, toxicity in animal studies indicates avoidance in early pregnancy
Breastfeeding	excreted in small amounts but no risk from therapeutic doses

References

ASTRA PHARMACEUTICALS LTD ™ – data sheets for XYLOCAINE ® (1990, 1995) and MARCAIN ® (1993)

Bevis, R. (1993). 'Obstetric anaesthesia and operations'. In: Bennett, V.R., Brown, L.K. (Eds). *Myles Textbook For Midwives.* 12th ed. Chapter 28, pp. 441–461. Edinburgh: Churchill Livingstone.

Briggs, G.G., Freeman, R.K., Yaffe, S.J. (1990). *Drugs In Pregnancy And Lactation: A Reference Guide To Fetal And Neonatal Risk.* 3rd edition. Baltimore: Williams and Wilkins.

Hopkins, S.J. (1995). *Drugs And Pharmacology For Nurses.* 12th ed. Edinburgh: Churchill Livingstone.

British Medical Association and the Royal Pharmaceutical Society of Great Britain (1996). *British National Formulary.* No. 31, March, Avon: Bath Press.

Department of Health et al (1996). *Report On The Confidential Enquiries Into Maternal Deaths In The United Kingdom 1991–93.* London: HMSO.

Further reading and research

Bevis, R. (1984). *Anaesthesia In Midwifery.* London: Bailliere Tindall.

Dennis, A.R., Leeson-Payne, C.G., Langham, B.T., Aitkenhead, A.R. (1995). 'Local anaesthesia for cannulation: Has practice changed'. *Anaesthesia,* Vol. 50, pp. 400–402.

Mahajan, J., Mahajan, R.P., Singh, M.M. et al (1993). 'Anaesthetic technique for elective casarean section and neurobehavioural status of the newborn'. *International Journal Of Obstetric Anaesthesia,* Vol. 2, No. 2, April, pp. 89–93.

Sepkoski, C.M., Lester, B.M., Ostheimer, G.W., Brazleton, T.B. (1992). 'The effects of maternal epidural anaesthesia on neonatal behaviour during the first month'. *Developmental Medicine And Child Neurology,* No. 34, pp. 1072–1080.

Enkin, M., Kierse, M., Renfrew, M., Neilsson, J. (1995). *A Guide To Effective Care In Pregnancy And Childbirth.* 2nd ed. Chapter 47. pp. 364–370.

Vamer, R.G. (1993). 'Mechanisms of regurgitation and its prevention with cricoid pressure'. *International Journal Of Obstetrical Anaesthesia,* Vol. 2, No. 4, October pp. 207–215.

With thanks to Richard Foxall MD Consultant Anaesthetist at West Dorset General Hospital, Dorchester for his help in compiling this chapter.

CHAPTER THREE

Analgesics

These preparations are used to relieve pain without causing unconsciousness or lack of all nervous sensation in a particular area. It is important to become familiar with pain theories and to use the body's natural analgesics to their optimum effect, as well as using chemical preparations.

The student should be aware of:

• pain theories, especially the 'gate theory' of Melzack and Wall (1964),

• the difference between anaesthesia and analgesia,

• the accumulative effect of many analgesics which can lead to intentional or accidental overdose,

• the different combinations of separate analgesic compounds,

• the possibility of addiction to analgesics,

• neonatal sequelae to maternal analgesia and

• the appropriateness of analgesic compound to complaint.

B.P.	diamorphine hydrochloride
Proprietary	aka HEROIN
Group	analgesic – morphine salt – narcotic
Uses/indications	moderate to severe pain, i.e. post operative and labour
Type of drug	CD, Class A, Schedule 2
Presentation	tablets, powder for reconstitution, linctus
Dosage	5–10 mg 4 hrly (dependent on patient size), 3 mg in 5 ml of linctus
Route of admin.	IM, oral
Contra-ind.	existing respiratory depression, asthma, raised intracranial pressure as it affects papillary responses
Side effects	sedation, nausea, vomiting, respiratory depression, dependence, tachycardia, hypothermia, hallucinations, mood swings, facial flushing, sweating, constipation
Interactions	*alcohol* – enhances the sedative effect, increases hypotension *antidepressants* – avoid concurrent administration of MAOI or administration within 2 weeks of their discontinuation *anxiolytics and hypnotics* – enhances the sedative effect
Fetal risk	crosses the placental barrier within 1 hour of administration, causes withdrawal symptoms, respiratory depression, meconium aspiration, intrauterine death
Breastfeeding	therapeutic doses unlikely to affect infant but in dependent mothers it is secreted into the breastmilk and causes addiction

B.P.	morphine sulphate
Proprietary	
Group	analgesic – narcotic
Uses/indications	post operative pain, intracathecal in epidurals in very small doses
Type of drug	CD, Class A, Schedule 2
Presentation	oral solution, tablets, suspension, ampoules
Dosage	10–15 mg 4 hrly
Route of admin.	oral, IM, s.c., p.r., IV, intracathecal
Contra-ind.	renal or hepatic impaitment, respiratory depression, asthma, raised intracranial pressure (affects papillary responses)
Side effects	respiratory depression, nausea, vomiting, confusion, dependence, constipation, hypothermia, postural hypotension, difficulty with micturition
Interactions	as for diamorphine
Fetal risk	as for diamorphine
Breastfeeding	as for diamorphine

B.P.	pethidine hydrochloride
Proprietary	PETHIDINE ®, PAMERGAN P100 ®
Group	analgesic – opioid, alkaloid
Uses/indications	moderate to severe pain, obstetric analgesia
Type of drug	CD, Class A, Schedule 2, authorized by standing orders
Presentation	tablets, ampoules
Dosage	*oral* – 50–100 mg 4 hrly *s.c./IM* – 25–150 mg 4 hrly *IV* – 25–50 mg 4 hrly
Route of admin.	oral, s.c., IM, IV
Contra-ind.	existing respiratory depression, renal impairment, pre-existing morphine addiction, compromised fetus
Side effects	nausea, vomiting, respiratory depression, convulsions after overdose, bradycardia, dependance
Interactions	as for diamorphine, *antacids* – cimetidine inhibits metabolism of pethidine
Fetal risk	crosses placental barrier within 2 minutes of administration and present in amniotic fluid in 30 mins, bradycardia, respiratory depression, withdrawal symptoms, slow excretion by neonatal liver
Breastfeeding	depresses suck reflex, as for diamorphine

B.P.	fentanyl
Proprietary	SUBLIMAZE ®, FENTANYL CITRATE ®,
Group	analgesic, opioid – morphine salt
Uses/indications	enhancement of anaesthesia i.e. epidural
Type of drug	CD, Class A, Schedule 2
Presentation	pre-diluted ampoules
Dosage	50–200 µg, subsequent doses 50 ug p.r.n.
Route of admin.	IV or intracathecal
Contra-ind.	caution in existing respiratory depression, myasthenia gravis
Side effects	respiratory depression, transient hypotension, bradycardia, nausea, vomiting, itching
Interactions	as for morphine
Fetal risk	can cause loss of fetal heart variability without fetal hypoxia, respiratory depression, withdrawal symptoms
Breastfeeding	no data available

B.P.	dihydrocodeine tartrate
Proprietary	DF118 ®, DHC CONTINUS ®, DIHYDROCODEINE
Group	analgesic, opioid – morphine salt
Uses/indications	moderate to severe pain
Type of drug	PoM, CD
Presentation	tablets (white), elixir, ampoules (CD)
Dosage	*oral* – 30 mg 4–6 hrly (preferably after food), higher doses causes nausea and vomiting *IM* – 50 mg 4–6 hrly
Route of admin.	oral, IM, deep s.c.
Contra-ind.	raised intracranial pressure, respiratory difficulties
Side effects	constipation, drowsiness, respiratory depression, hypotension, dizziness, dependance, high doses cause nausea and vomiting
Interactions	as for diamorphine
Fetal risk	withdrawal symptoms, respiratory depression in the neonate
Breastfeeding	no data available

B.P.	codeine phosphate
Proprietary	
Group	analgesic, opioid – morphine salt
Uses/indications	mild to moderate pain
Type of drug	PoM, CD
Presentation	tablets, syrup, ampoules (CD)
Dosage	*oral* – 30–60 mg 4 hrly (240 mg daily max.) *IM* – 30–60 mg 4 hrly
Route of admin.	oral, IM
Contra-ind.	raised intracranial pressure
Side effects	constipation, nausea, sedation, respiratory depression, especially cough reflex, dependence
Interactions	as for diamorphine
Fetal risk	*1st trimester* – inguinal hernias, cardiac and circulatory system defects, cleft lip and palate *2nd trimester* – alimentary tract defects *labour* – neonatal respiratory depression and withdrawal
Breastfeeding	amount secreted too small to be harmful

B.P.	aspirin (acetylsalicyclic acid)
Proprietary	CAPRIN ®, NU-SEALS ®, ASPRO ®, ASPRO-CLEAR ® (refer to pharmacist for advice)
Group	analgesic, non-opioid, NSAID
Uses/indications	mild to moderate pain, pyrexia
Type of drug	GSL
Presentation	tablets (pink, red or white), some dispersible
Dosage	1200 mg – 4 g daily (evenly divided doses)
Route of admin.	oral
Contra-ind.	gastric ulceration, asthma, pregnancy unless in very low doses under obstetricians orders
Side effects	gastric irritation/ulceration, increased bleeding time leading to haemorrhage i.e. aph, iph, pph, delayed onset and duration or labour (low doses are not harmful), bronchospasm and skin reactions in hyper-sensitive patients.
Interactions	*antacids* – increased alkalinity of urine *analgesics* – concommitant admin. increases side effects *anticoagulants* – increased risk of haemorrhage (potentiates antiplatelet effect) *antiepileptics* – enhance effect of phenytoin and valporate
Fetal risk	in high doses closure of PDA *in utero,* persistent pulmonary hypertension, kernicterus in jaundiced neonates, is also reported to be linked with fetal growth deficiency, and a purpuric rash in neonates with depression of the platelet function
Breastfeeding	potentially Reyes Syndrome, impairment of platelet function and hypoprothrombiaemia if neonatal vitamin K stores are low

B.P.	diclofenac sodium
Proprietary	VOLTAROL ®
Group	analgesic, non-opioid, NSAID
Uses/indications	moderate to severe pain, musculo-skeletal pain, used post LSCS, anti-inflammatory properties
Type of drug	PoM
Presentation	tablets (brown), ampoules, suppositories
Dosage	*oral* – 75–150 mg daily in divided doses preferably after food *deep IM* – 75 mg daily (max. 2 days) *p.r.* – 100 mg 18 hrly
Route of admin.	oral, deep IM, p.r.
Contra-ind.	asthma, pregnancy
Side effects	delayed onset and increased duration of labour, gastric irritability/ulceration, coagulation disorders leading to haemorrhage, headache, dizziness, vertigo
Interactions	*analgesics* – concommitant admin. causes increased side effects *antihypertensives* – increased hypertensive effects *beta-blockers* – antagonism of hypertensive effects
Fetal risk	can cause closure of PDA *in utero*, persistent pulmonary hypertension
Breastfeeding	amount secreted too small to be harmful

B.P.	paracetamol
Proprietary	PANADOL ®, CALPOL ® (refer to pharmacist for advice)
Group	analgesic, non-opioid
Uses/indications	mild to moderate pain, pyrexia
Type of drug	GSL
Presentation	tablets, oral suspension, dispersible tablets, suppositories
Dosage	500 mg–1 g 4–6 hrly (max. 4 g daily)
Route of admin.	oral, p.r.
Contra-ind.	hepatic and renal disease, alcohol dependence
Side effects	*rare,* blood disorders, rashes, overdose causes liver damage
Interactions	*anticoagulants* – with prolonged use seems to enhance effect of warfarin
Fetal risk	no data available
Breastfeeding	short courses only – amount secreted too small to be harmful

B.P.	ibuprofen
Proprietary	BRUFEN ®, (GSL - NUROFEN ®)
Group	analgesic, non-opioid, NSAID
Uses/indications	mild to moderate pain, particularly perineal
Type of drug	PoM, GSL
Presentation	tablets, syrup, granules
Dosage	1.2–1.8 g daily in 3–4 doses (after food)
Route of admin.	oral
Contra-ind.	pregnancy, salicyclate hypersensitivity, asthma
Side effects	gastro-intestinal discomfort, diarrhoea, nausea, rash, headache, dizziness
Interactions	as for diclofenac
Fetal risk	as for salicyclic acid
Breastfeeding	apparently safe

B.P.	mefanamic acid
Proprietary	PONSTAN ®
Group	analgesic, non-opioid, NSAID
Uses/indications	mild to moderate pain, anti-inflammatory
Type of drug	PoM
Presentation	tablets (yellow), capsules (ivory/blue)
Dosage	500 mg t.d.s. after food
Route of admin.	oral
Contra-ind.	as for salicyclic acid
Side effects	drowsiness, diarrhoea, nausea, rash, thrombocytopenia, if these occur withdraw the drug
Interactions	as for diclofenac
Fetal risk	as for salicyclic acid
Breastfeeding	insufficient information to allow breastfeeding safely

B.P.	co-codamol (paracetamol 500 mg + codeine 8 mg)
Proprietary	SOLPADOL ®, TYLEX ® (paracetamol 500 mg + codeine 30 mg)
Group	analgesic, non-opioid
Uses/indications	mild to moderate pain
Type of drug	PoM (30/500), GSL (8/500)
Presentation	tablets, capsules, dispersible tablets
Dosage	1–2 tablets or capsules 4 hrly, max. 8 daily
Route of admin.	oral
Contra-ind.	as for paracetamol and for codeine
Side effects	as for paracetamol and codeine phosphate
Interactions	as for paracetamol and codeine phosphate
Fetal risk	as for codeine phosphate
Breastfeeding	amount secreted too small to be harmful

B.P	codydramol (pararcetamol 500 mg + dihydrocodiene 10 mg)
Proprietary	PARAMOL ®
Group	analgesic, paracetamol and opioid compound
Uses/indications	mild to moderate pain
Type of drug	PoM
Presentation	tablets (white)
Dosage	1–2 tablets 4–6 hrly (max 8 daily)
Route of admin.	oral
Contra-ind.	as for paracetamol and dihydrocodeine
Side effects	as for paracetamol and dihydrocodeine
Interactions	as for paracetamol and dihydrocodeine
Fetal risk	as for dihydrocodeine
Breastfeeding	no data available

B.P	co-proxamol (paracetamol 325 mg + dextropropoxyphene 32.5mg)
Proprietary	DISTALGESIC ®
Group	analgesic, compound of paracetamol and opioid salt
Uses/indications	mild to moderate pain
Type of drug	PoM, GSL
Presentation	tablets (white)
Dosage	1–2 tablets 4-6 hrly (max. 8 daily)
Route of admin.	oral
Contra-ind.	alcohol abuse
Side effects	action is similar to codeine and therefore has similar effect, overdose is complicated by respiratory depression, heart failure and by hepatic failure
Interactions	*anticoagulant* – effect of warfarin possibly enhanced
Fetal risk	as for codeine
Breastfeeding	amount secreted too small to be harmful

B.P.	co-codaprin (aspirin 400 mg/ codeine phosphate 8 mg)
Proprietary	
Group	analgesic, aspirin compound
Uses/indications	mild to moderate pain
Type of drug	PoM
Presentation	tablets (white)
Dosage	1–2 tablets 4–6 hrly (max. 8 daily)
Route of admin.	oral
Contra-ind.	as for codeine and aspirin
Side effects	as for codeine and aspirin
Interactions	as for codeine and aspirin
Fetal risk	as for codeine and aspirin
Breastfeeding	should be avoided in view of aspirin content

References

Bevis, R. (1993). 'Pain relief and comfort in labour'. In: Bennett, V.R., Brown, L.K. (Eds). *Myles Textbook For Midwives*, 12th edition. Chapter 13, pp. 184–198. Edinburgh: Churchill Livingstone.

Briggs, G.G., Freeman, R.K., Yaffe, S.J. (1990). *Drugs In Pregnancy And Lactation: A Reference Guide To Fetal And Neonatal Risk*. 3rd edition. Baltimore: Williams and Wilkins.

British Medical Association and the Royal Pharmaceutical Society of Great Britain (1996). *British National Formulary*. No. 31, March, Avon: Bath Press.

EVANS ™ – data sheets – DIAMORPHINE (1996)

Hopkins, S.J. (1995). *Drugs And Pharmacology For Nurses*. 12th edition. Edinburgh: Churchill Livingstone.

Niven, C. (1994). 'Coping with labour pain, the midwifes role'. In: Robinson, S., Thompson, A.M. (Eds). *Midwives, Research And Childbirth*. Vol 3. Chapter 5, pp. 91–119. London: Chapman and Hall.

Read, M.D., Golightly, P.W, Grant, E. (1996). *Drugs In Breast Milk*. 14th edition. Boehringer Ingelheim Ltd

Further reading

Yerby, M. (1996). 'Managing pain in labour Pt 2 Non-pharmacological pain relief'. *Modern Midwife*, Vol. 6, No. 4, April, pp. 16–18.

Yerby, M. (1996). 'Managing pain in labour Pt 3 Pharmacological methods of pain relief'. *Modern Midwife*, Vol. 6, No. 5, May, pp. 22–25.

CHAPTER FOUR

Antibiotics

These are substances which are produced by certain bacteria or fungi which interfere with or prevent the growth of other bacteria/fungi. They are used in infection or as prophylaxis e.g. in cases of spontaneous rupture of membranes longer than 24 hours or lower segment caesarean section.

The student should be aware of:

- causes and transmission of infection,

- causal organisms of infection and their laboratory identification,

- symptoms and progression of infection,

- the importance of bacterial culture and sensitivity,

- the ingestion, uptake, action and excretion of the drug prescribed and

- the risk of candida infection as a result of antibiotic therapy.

B.P.	**amoxycillin**
Proprietary	AMOXIL ®, ALMODAN ®
Group	antibiotics, penicillin
Uses/indications	broad spectrum, gram-ve except pseudomonas, respiratory infections, UTI, gonorrhoea
Type of drug	PoM
Presentation	capsules (maroon/gold), dispersible tablets, sachets, powder for reconstitution
Dosage	*oral* – 250–500 mg t.d.s. *IM* – 750–1500 mg daily *IV* – 500 mg t.d.s. to 1 g q.d.s. in severe infection
Route of admin.	oral, IM, IV/infusion
Contra-ind.	penicillin hypersensitivity
Side effects	mild diarrhoea, indigestion, rash, thrush
Interactions	*contraceptives* – reduces contraceptive effect *uricosurics* – excretion reduced with concommitant admin. of probenecid – used in treatment of gonorrhoea
Fetal risk	nil known, no reports of toxicity in animal or human studies
Breastfeeding	considered safe but modifies the bowel flora and can cause sensitization and interferes with culture results if an infection screen is required

B.P.	co-amoxiclav (compound of amoxycillin as a sodium salt and clavunic acid)
Proprietary	AUGMENTIN ®
Group	antibiotic, penicillin, broad spectrum
Uses/indications	against bacteria resistant to amoxycillin, i.e. staph. aureus, E-coli, gonorrhoea
Type of drug	PoM
Presentation	tablets (white ovals), dispersible tablets, suspension, powder for reconstitution
Dosage	*oral* – 375 mg (250 mg expressed as amoxycillin) t.d.s., 625 mg (500 mg) t.d.s. in severe infection *IV* – 1–2 g t.d.s.
Route of admin.	oral, IV, IV infusion
Contra-ind.	penicillin hypersensitivity
Side effects	nausea, diarrhoea, rashes, rarely hepatic impairment, hypersensitivity
Interactions	*anticoagulants* – may prolong bleeding time and prothrombin time *contraceptives* – reduces contraceptive effect
Fetal risk	animal studies with oral and parenteral administration show no teratogenicity but manufacturers advise avoidance in the first trimester and thereafter only when considered essential
Breastfeeding	considered safe but as for amoxycillin

B.P.	flucloxacillin sodium
Proprietary	FLOXAPEN ®, LADROPEN ®, STAFOXIL ®, STAPHILPEN ®
Group	antibiotic, penicillinase resistant penicillin
Uses/indications	against beta-lactamase resistant microbes e.g. staph. aureus, prophylaxis in surgery
Type of drug	PoM
Presentation	capsules (black/caramel), syrup, powder for reconstitution
Dosage	*oral* – 250 mg t.d.s. (30 mins before food) *IV/infusion* – 250 mg–1g t.d.s. *IM* – 250 mg q.d.s. (dosage may be doubled in severe infection)
Route of admin.	oral, IM, IV/infusion
Contra-ind.	penicillin hypersensitivity
Side effects	diarrhoea, rash, indigestion, rarely hepatic impairment
Interactions	*contraceptives* – reduces contraceptive effect
Fetal risk	animal studies show no teratogenicity but manufacturer advises that it should be withheld unless considered essential
Breastfeeding	considered safe, but as for amoxycillin

B.P.	cephradine
Proprietary	VELOSEF ®
Group	antibiotic - cephalosporin
Uses/indications	against both gram +ve and -ve bacteria, prophylaxis with LSCS
Type of drug	PoM
Presentation	capsules (blue), syrup, powder for reconstitution
Dosage	*oral* – 250–500 mg 6–8 hrly *IM/IV* – 500 mg – 1g q.d.s.
Route of admin.	oral, IM, IV
Contra-ind.	renal dysfunction
Side effects	nausea, diarrhoea and hypersensitivity
Interactions	*anticoagulants* – effect of warfarin enhanced *uricosurics* – excretion is reduced by probenecid
Fetal risk	no reports of congenital defects located
Breastfeeding	considered safe but as for amoxycillin

B.P.	erythromycin
Proprietary	ERYTHROCIN ®, ERYCEN ®, ERYTHROPED ®, ILOSONE ®
Group	antibiotic, macrolide
Uses/indications	penicillin resisitant organisms, syphilis, chlamydia, respiratory infection
Type of drug	PoM
Presentation	tablets, capsules, powder for reconstitution, granules, suspension
Dosage	*oral* – 250–500 mg q.d.s. or 0.5–1 g b.d. syphilis 500 mg q.d.s. for 14 days *IV* – 25–50 mg/kg daily
Route of admin.	oral, IV
Contra-ind.	hypersensitivity, hepatic dysfunction
Side effects	nausea, vomiting, fever skin eruptions, urticaria, rashes, in large doses – reversible hearing loss, hepatic dysfunction, thrombophlebitis following IV
Interactions	*anticoagulants* – effect of warfarin enhanced *antihistamines* – inhibits the metabolism of terfenadine causing dangerous arrhythmias *ergotamines* – ergotism reported *theophylline* – inhibition of metabolism of theophylline
Fetal risk	no reports of congenital defects located
Breastfeeding	only secreted in small amounts in breastmilk – as for amoxycillin

B.P.	metronidazole
Proprietary	FLAGYL ®,ZADSTADT ®, METROLYL ®, NIDAZOL ®
Group	antibiotic
Uses/indications	anaerobes, prophylaxis in surgery, clostridium, trichomonas vaginalis
Type of drug	PoM
Presentation	tablets (ivory), suspension
Dosage	*oral* – stat 800 mg then 400 mg t.d.s. *IV* – 500 mg t.d.s. LSCS 400 mg t.d.s. (500 mg at intubation)
Route of admin.	oral, p.r., IV
Contra-ind.	in pregnancy and breastfeeding avoid high dosage, avoid alcohol
Side effects	unpleasant taste in mouth, furry tongue, nausea, vomiting, rashes, headache, drowsiness, dizziness
Interactions	*alcohol* – disufilram like reaction *anticoagulants* – enhances the effect of warfarin *antiepileptics* – inhibits the metabolism of phenytoin phenobarbitone accelerates metabolism of metronidazole
Fetal risk	avoid high dose regimens, can cause midline facial defects, cardiac defects, genital defects and limb defects
Breastfeeding	significant amounts secreted, avoid large single doses

References

BEECHAM RESEARCH™ – data sheets – AUGMENTIN ®, FLOXAPEN ®

Briggs, G.G., Freeman, R.K., Yaffe, S.J. (1990). *Drugs in Pregnancy and Lactation: A Reference Guide to Fetal and Neonatal Risk.* 3rd edition. Baltimore: Williams and Wilkins.

British Medical Association and the Royal Pharmaceutical Society of Great Britain (1996). *British National Formulary.* No. 31, March, Avon: Bath Press.

Hopkins, S.J. (1995). *Drugs and Pharmocology for Nurses.* 12th edition. Edinburgh: Churchill Livingstone.

Read, M.D., Golightly, P.W., Grant, E. (1996). *Drugs in Breast Milk.* 14th edition. Boehringer Ingelheim Ltd

RHONE-POULENC AND RORER ™ – data sheets – FLAGYLL ®

Roth, C. (1993). 'Genital and sexually transmissable infections in pregnancy'. In: Bennett, V.R., Brown, L.K. (Eds). *Myles Textbook for Midwives.* 12th edition. Edinburgh: Churchill Livingstone. Chapter 19, pp. 284–305.

Further reading

Enkin, M., Kierse, M., Renfrew, M., Neilsson, J. (1995). *A Guide To Effective Care In Pregnancy And Childbirth.* 2nd edition. Oxford: Oxford University Press.

Kenyon, S. (1995). 'O.R.A.C.L.E. - An overview of the evidence'. *MIDIRS Midwifery Digest,* Vol. 5, No. 1, March, pp. 14–16.

CHAPTER FIVE

Anticoagulants

These are substances used to prevent blood clotting.

The student should be aware of:

- factors predisposing to thromboembolism,

- local protocols for management of thromboembolism,

- the antagonist for such treatment and its availability,

- factors involved in the mechanism of blood clotting,

- conditions requiring treatment with anticoagulants,

- maternal and fetal sequelae of such treatment and

- the effects of progesterone on the circulatory system.

B.P.	heparin (as sodium or calcium salt)
Proprietary	CALCIPRINE ®, MONOPARIN ®, MINIHEP ®, UNIHEP ®, DALTEPARIN ®
Group	anticoagulant, parenteral
Uses/indications	treatment of DVT, pulmonary embolism, thromboembolic susceptible clients
Type of drug	PoM
Presentation	preloaded syringes, ampoules
Dosage	*IV* – 5000 units loading dose and then continuous confusion of 1000–2000 units/hr adjusted by laboratory monitoring. *s.c.* – 5000 8–12 hrly until ambulant *pregnancy* – 10,000 units 12 hrly *DVT* – 10–20,000 units 12 hrly
Route of admin.	s.c., IV
Contra-ind.	haemorrhagic disorders, cerebral aneurysm, severe hypertension
Side effects	haemorrhage including placental sites, thrombocytopenia, hypersensitivity, bruising and haematoma formation
Interactions	*aspirin* – antiplatelet effect enhanced by heparin
Fetal risk	available data suggests there is no risk to fetus or neonate
Breastfeeding	not excreted in breastmilk
Antagonist	**protamine sulphate**

The dosage of *heparin* in prophylaxis will vary according to individual circumstances, and the opinion of the haematologist and medical physician treating the client in conjunction with the obstetric team.

B.P.	warfarin sodium
Proprietary	MAREVAN ®, WARFARIN WBP ®
Group	anticoagulant – oral
Uses/indications	prophylaxis after prosthetic heart valve surgery, DVT, pulmonary embolism
Type of drug	PoM
Presentation	tablets: brown – 1 mg, blue – 3 mg, pink – 5mg
Dosage	refer to pharmacist or BNF, usually 3–10 mg daily
Route of admin.	oral
Contra-ind.	*pregnancy*, but may be used between 16–36 weeks gestation if heparin not available and risks of thrombosis outweigh the risk to the fetus
Side effects	haemorrhage, nausea, transient alopecia
Fetal risk	fetal teratogen, should stopped pre-conception or within 6 week gestation, haemorrhage in fetus and placenta
Interactions	*alcohol* – enhanced effects with large alcohol doses *antacids* – cimtetidine inhibits the metabolism and enhances the effect of warfarin *aspirin* – increased risk of haemorrhage *erythromycin and metronidazole* – enhance effects of warfarin *paracetamol* – theoretical increased risk of bleeds *phenobarbitone* – diminishes warfarins effects

	phenytoin – both enhances and diminishes warfarins effect *oral contraceptive* – diminished contraceptive effect
Breastfeeding	not excreted in breastmilk, theoretical risk of haemorrhage especially with Vitamin K deficiency
Antagonist	**Vitamin K and plasma**

The dosage of *warfarin* in prophylaxis will vary according to individual circumstances, and the opinion of the haematologist and medical physician treating the client in conjunction with the obstetric team.

B.P.	protamine sulphate
Proprietary	
Group	anticoagulant, ANTAGONIST
Uses/indications	antagonist to heparin
Type of drug	PoM
Presentation	ampoules
Dosage	1 mg neutralizes 100 units heparin (mucous) or 80 units (lung) within 15 minutes of heparin administration, if longer less is required as heparin is rapidly excreted. Max. dose 50 mg in 10 minutes. Should be monitored by Activated Partial Prothrombin Time (APPT) or other clotting test
Route of admin.	slow IV
Contra-ind.	hypersensitivity to protamine, caution in those receiving protamine insulin preparation i.e. isophane insulin
Side effects	flushing, hypotension, bradycardia, if overdosed then acts as an anticoagulant
Interactions	caution in those receiving isophane insulins – hypersensitivity
Fetal risk	insufficient information available – no animal or human studies have been carried out.
Breastfeeding	no data available – as for fetal risk

B.P.	**phytomendione (Vitamin K)**
Proprietary	KONAKION ®
Group	anticoagulant – ANTAGONIST
Uses/indications	prevention and treatment of haemorrhage
Type of drug	PoM
Presentation	tablets, ampoules
Dosage	*life threatening haemorrhage* – 5 mg slow IV injection plus plasma (factors II, IX, VII if available) *less severe haemorrhage* – withold warfarin and consider 0.5–2 mg slow IV injection
Route of admin.	very slow IV injection, oral, IM
Contra-ind.	no data available
Side effects	no data available
Interactions	nil recorded
Fetal risk	poor placental transfer, no risk data available
Breastfeeding	maternal doses – not enough information available to allow classification as safe drug large maternal doses of anticoagulants may require neonatal Vitamin K prophylaxis

References

Ball, J.A. (1993). 'Complications of the puerperium'. In: Bennett, V.R., Brown, L.K. (Eds). *Myles Textbook For Midwives*. 12th edition Chapter 30, pp. 483–486. Edinburgh: Churchill Livingstone.

Briggs, G.G., Freeman, R.K., Yaffe, S.J. (1990). *Drugs In Pregnancy And Lactation: A Reference Guide To Fetal And Neonatal Risk*. 3rd edition. Baltimore: Williams and Wilkins.

British Medical Association and the Royal Pharmaceutical Society of Great Britain (1996). *British National Formulary*. No. 31, March, Avon: Bath Press.

EVANS ™ – Summary of Product Characteristics (SPC) – Protamine Sulphate.

Hopkins, S.J. (1995). *Drugs And Phamacology For Nurses* 12th edition. Edinburgh: Churchill Livingstone.

Read, M.W., Golightly, P.W., Grant, E. (1996). *Drugs In Breast Milk*. 14th edition. Boehringer Ingelheim Ltd.

CHAPTER SIX

Anticonvulsants

These are drugs used to arrest or prevent fits or seizures. The benefits of treatment should outweigh the risk to the fetus and efforts should be made to use the single most effective drug as teratogenicity increases with the number of drugs used.

This drug group inhibits the uptake of folic acid and therefore any supplements given may need to be continued throughout pregnancy.

Magnesium sulphate is also an anticonvulsant used in the emergency treatment of eclampsia (see Chapter 25 on emergency drugs).

The student should be aware of:

- conditions which require anticonvulsant therapy,

- local protocols for anticonvulsant therapy,

- recognition of fits, seizures and convulsions,

- resuscitative techniques and care of affected clients and

- maternal and fetal sequelae of absorption of these preparations.

B.P.	phenytoin
Proprietary	EPANUTIN ®
Group	anticonvulsant/antiepileptic
Uses/indications	epilepsy, fits not absence seizures, treatment of eclampsia
Type of drug	PoM, Class 1
Presentation	capsules, tablets, suspension
Dosage	*with or after food* – 150–300 mg/day in 1–2 divided doses or as per protocol (plasma values need evaluation and observation) *IV* – phenytoin sodium in treatment of eclampsia as per protocol
Route of admin.	oral, IV
Contra-ind.	*pregnancy* and *breastfeeding*
Side effects	nausea, vomiting, headache, tremor, insomnia *prolonged usage* – hirsutism, coarse facies, acne, gingival hyperplasia
Interactions	see end of chapter
Fetal risk	in trimesters 1 and 3 teratogen, maternal folic acid supplements should be given under medical supervision, increased risk of haemorrhage in the neonate prophylaxis with Vitamin K recommended
Breastfeeding	secreted in breast milk, some minor effects noted, mother and child should be monitored

B.P.	phenobarbitone
Proprietary	GARDENAL SODIUM ®
Group	antiepileptic – barbiturate
Uses/indications	epilepsy – not absence seizures, status epilepticus
Type of drug	PoM, CD
Presentation	tablets, elixir, ampoules
Dosage	*oral* – 50–200 mg q.d.s. to a max. 600 mg/day *IM* – 50–200 mg q.d.s. to a max. 600 mg/day (plasma monitoring is less useful as tolerance occurs)
Route of admin.	oral, IM, IV injection
Contra-ind.	pregnancy, breastfeeding, impaired hepatic function
Side effects	tolerance develops, drowsiness, neural depression, allergic skin reactions, overdose
Interactions	see end of chapter
Fetal risk	in trimesters 1 and 3 teratogen, hypoprothrombinaemia and withdrawal in infants with maternal treatment late in pregnancy, concomittant administration with other antiepileptics has been linked to haemorrhagic disease of the newborn within the first 24 hrs of life
Breastfeeding	avoid where possible, drowsiness in infant and other minor effects reported. Mother and baby need to be monitored

B.P.	sodium valproate
Proprietary	EPILIM ®
Group	anticonvulsant
Uses/indications	all forms of epilepsy, absence seizures
Type of drug	PoM
Presentation	tablets, solution, syrup
Dosage	oral – 600 mg–2.5 g/day
Route of admin.	oral
Contra-ind.	*pregnancy* and *breastfeeding*
Side effects	nausea, weight gain, hair loss, hepatic impairment, platelet function disturbed, multiple therapy requires care
Interactions	see end of chapter
Fetal risk	spina bifida, neonatal bleeding, hepatotoxicity, fetal growth deficiency, hyperbilirubinaemia, fetal distress, craniofacial defects, urogential defects, hyperspadias up to 50%, retarded psychomoter development, digit abnormalities
Breastfeeding	secreted in breast milk – in low doses appears safe high doses – insufficient information to qualify as safe

Interactions

Phenytoin

- analgesics – aspirin increases the plasma-phenytoin concentration.
- antacids – reduce the absorption of phenytoin.
- antibiotics – metronidazole increases the plasma phenytoin concentration.
- plasma concentration and antifoliate effect increased by trimoxazole and trimethoprim.
- anticoagulants – probably reduce the effect of warfarin.
- antiepileptics – two or more antiepilaeptics enhance toxicity, monitoring of plasma concentrations required.
- antiemetics – stemetil and derivatives lower convulsive threshold.
- antihypertensives – nifedipine increases phenytoin plasma concentration, the effect of nifedipine is reduced.
- anxiolytics and hypnotics – diazepam can increase or decrease plasma phenytoin concentration.
- corticosteroids – metabolism is increased therefore effect is decreased.
- contraceptives – metabolism of oral contraceptives is increased therefore their effect is decreased.
- vitamins – the plasma phenytoin concentration is lowered by folic acid, Vitamin D supplements may be required.

Phenobarbitone

- antibiotics – metabolism of metronidazole is increased therefore the effect is decreased.
- anticoagulants – metabolism of warfarin increased therefore effect decreased.
- antiepileptics – as for phenytoin, requires dose monitoring.
- antiemetics – as for phenytoin.
- antihypertensives – effect of nifedipine reduced.
- corticosteroids – as for phenytoin.
- contraceptives – as for phenytoin.

Sodium valproate

- analgesics – aspirin enhances effect.
- antiemetics – as for phenytoin.
- antiepileptics – with two or more, close monitoring is required.

References

Briggs, G.G., Freeman, R.K., Yaffe, S.J. (1990). *Drugs In Pregnancy And Lactation: A Reference Guide To Fetal And Neonatal Risk.* 3rd edition. Baltimore: Williams and Wilkins.

British Medical Association and Royal Pharmaceutical Society of Great Britain (1996). *British National Formulary.* No. 31, March, Avon: Bath Press.

Hopkins, S.J. (1995). *Drugs And Pharmacology For Nurses.* 12th edition. Edinburgh: Churchill Livingstone.

LLoyd, C., Lewis, V. (1993). 'Diseases associated with pregnancy'. In: Bennett, V.R., Brown, L.K. (Eds). *Myles Textbook For Midwives.* 12th edition. Chapter 22, pp. 362–363 Edinburgh: Churchill Livingstone.

RHONE - POULENC AND RORER™ – data sheets – GARDENAL ®

Read, M.D., Golightly, P.W., Grant, E. (1996). *Drugs In Breast Milk.* 14th edition, Boehringer Ingelheim Ltd.

CHAPTER SEVEN

Antidepressants

These are substances which aim to restore the balance of neurotransmitter substances in the brain, a deficiency of which is thought to contribute to depression. They are usually MonoAmine Oxidase Inhibitors (MAOIs) or tricyclic antidepressants.

The student should be aware of:

- the clinical signs and progression of ante and postnatal depression,

- the maternal and fetal sequelae of therapy,

- the local availability of counselling and facilities for treatment and

- the consequences for lack of either diagnosis or treatment of depression.

The author recommends that drugs in this group should be individually investigated as psychiatry is a specialized field and most antidepressants require monitoring in pregnancy and breastfeeding.

B.P.	dothiepin hydrochloride
Proprietary	PROTHIADEN ®
Group	antidepressant – tricyclic
Uses/indications	depression where sedation is required i.e. postnatal depression
Type of drug	PoM
Presentation	capsules (red/brown), red tablets
Dosage	oral – 75 mg daily (divided or single) increased to 150–225 mg daily
Route of admin.	oral
Contra-ind.	recent myocardial infarction, mania
Side effects	dry mouth, sedation, blurred vision cardio vascular disturbances, blood sugar changes
Interactions	*alcohol* – avoid – enhanced sedative effect *antidepressants* – CNS excitation, hypertension with MAOIs – avoid for two weeks after stopping MAOI *antiepileptics* – convulsive threshold is lowered and tricyclic plasma concentration is lowered *antihistamines* – increased antimuscarinic and sedative effect, ventricular arrythmias with terfenadine and astemizole *antihypertensives* – increases hypotensive effect *contraceptives* – antagonizes effect of antidepressants but side effects increase the plasma concentration of tricyclics
Fetal risk	tachycardia, irritability, muscle spasms and neonatal convulsions
Breastfeeding	amount secreted too small to be harmful in short term use

References

Briggs, G.G., Freeman, R.K., Yaffe, S.J. (1990). *Drugs In Pregnancy And Lactation: A Reference Guide To Fetal And Neonatal Risk.* 3rd edition. Baltimore: Williams and Wilkins.

British Medical Association and Royal Pharmaceutical Society of Great Britain (1996). *British National Formulary.* No. 31, March, Avon: Bath Press.

Hopkins, S.J. (1995). *Drugs And Pharmacology For Nurses.* 12th edition, Edinburgh: Churchill Livingstone.

Read, M.D., Golightly, P.W., Grant, E. (1996). *Drugs In Breast Milk.* 14th edition. Boehringer Ingelheim Ltd

Further reading

Batagol, R. (1994). 'Antidepressant drugs and breast feeding'. *Australian Lactation Consultants Association News*, Vol. 5, No. 1, April, pp. 24–25. In: *MIDIRS Midwifery Digest,* September, Vol. 4, No. 3, pp. 346–347.

Berger, A. (1995). 'The danger of blues for a boy'. *New Scientist*, 8th July p.4.

Levy, V. (1994). 'The maternity blues in postpartum women and post-operative patients'. In: Robinson, S., Thompson, A.M. (Eds). *Midwives, Research And Childbirth*, Chapter 7, pp. 147–174. London: Chapman and Hall.

Small, R., Brown, S., Lumley, J. (1994). 'Missing voices: what women say and do about depression after childbirth'. *Journal Of Reproduction And Infant Psychology*, Vol. 12, No. 2, April-June, pp. 89–103.

CHAPTER EIGHT

Antiemetics

These are drugs used to prevent or lessen nausea and vomiting. Some of these preparations may also be antipsychotics or antihistamines.

The student should be aware of:

- the actions of analgesics on the cerebral cortex,

- the results of administration of the antipsychotic antiemetics i.e. their potentiating effects and

- the appropriateness of treatment using antiemetics especially in early pregnancy.

B.P.	metochlopromide hydrochloride
Proprietary	MAXOLON ®
Group	antiemetic
Uses/indications	nausea, vomiting
Type of drug	PoM
Presentation	tablets, ampoules, infusion, oral suspension
Dosage	15–30 mg daily
Route of admin.	IM, oral, IVI
Contra-ind.	hepatic and renal impairment, may cause hypertension in phaeochromocytoma
Side effects	extrapyramidial effects, hyperprolactinaemia
Interactions	*analgesics* – increases the absorption of aspirin and paracetamol therefore enhancing their effect opioid *analgesics* – antagonize the effect on gasto-intestinal activity
Fetal risk	use with caution, there is no information on the long term evaluation on infants exposed *in utero*
Breastfeeding	use with caution as there is a theoretical risk of potent central nervous system effects

B.P.	prochlorperazine
Proprietary	STEMETIL ®, BUCCASTEM ®
Group	antiemetic – antipsychotic
Uses/indications	prophylaxis with the use of opioid analgesic, with excessive emesis
Type of drug	PoM
Presentation	ampoules, tablets
Dosage	IM – 12.5 mg 6–8 hrly
Route of admin.	IM, oral
Contra-ind.	*pregnancy*, myasthenia gravis, cardio-vascular and respiratory disease, epilepsy, phaeochromocytoma
Side effects	can cause prolonged labour and should be withheld until 3–4 cm dilatation, drowsiness, pallor, hypothermia, extrapyramidal effects
Interactions	*alcohol* – increases the sedative effect *anaesthetics* – increases their hypotensive effect *antiepileptics* – lowers convulsive threshold *antihistamines* – increased risk of ventricular arrythmias with terfenadine *antihypertensives* – with methyldopa there is an increased risk of extrapyramidal effects
Fetal risk	in the first trimester there are reports of congenital defects associated with repeated use even at low doses, however single or occasional low doses appear safe. Extrapyramidal symptoms in the neonate, lethargy and tremor, low APGARs, paradoxical hyperexcitability
Breastfeeding	amount probably too small to be excreted but avoid unless absolutely necessary, the manufacturer recommends against therapy during breastfeeding

B.P.	**promazine hydrochloride**
Proprietary	SPARINE ®
Group	antiemetic – antipsychotic
Uses/indications	relaxant, antiemetic in conjunction with opioids
Type of drug	PoM
Presentation	ampoules
Dosage	50 mg 6–8 hrly
Route of admin.	IM
Contra-ind.	as for prochlorperazine
Side effects	drowsiness, amnesia, pallor, extrapyramidial symptoms
Interactions	as for prochlorperazine
Fetal risk	consensus of research reports no adverse effects but use with caution due to potential teratogenicity and central nervous system effects on the neonate
Breastfeeding	as for prochlorperazine – but the manufacturer recommends that the product should not be used in conjunction with breastfeeding

References

Briggs, G.G., Freeman, R.K., Yaffe, S.J. (1990). *Drugs In Pregnancy And Lactation: A Reference Guide To Fetal And Neonatal Risk.* 3rd edition. Baltimore: Williams and Wilkins.

British Medical Association and the Royal Pharmaceutical Society of Great Britain (1996). *British National Formulary.* No. 31, March, Avon: Bath Press.

Hopkins, S.J. (1995). *Drugs And Pharmacology For Nurses.* 12th edition. Edinburgh: Churchill Livingstone.

Read, M.D., Golightly, P.W., Grant, E. (1996). *Drugs In Breast Milk.* 14th ed. Boehringer Ingelheim Ltd

RHONE – POULENC AND RORER ™ – data sheets – STEMETIL ®

WYETH ™ – data sheets – SPARINE ®

CHAPTER NINE

Antihypertensives

These are substances used to control or modify blood pressure either by reducing peripheral resistance or blocking alpha or beta adrenoreceptors in the heart or by reducing the central flow of impulses to the sympathetic nerves and decreasing the release of noradrenaline at adrenogenic nerve endings.

The student should be aware of:

- the physiology and pathophysiology of blood pressure,

- the aetiology, pathophysiology and progression of pregnancy induced hypertension and pre-eclampsia,

- the difference between essential hypertension and pregnancy induced hypertension and pre-eclampsia/eclampsia,

- the maternal and fetal sequelae of therapy using these substances and

- the local protocols for treatment in cases of eclampsia (see emergency drugs).

B.P.	**hydrallazine hydrochloride**
Proprietary	HYDRALLAZINE, APRESOLINE ®
Group	antihypertensive – vasodilator
Uses/indications	raised diastolic blood pressure used concomitantly with other therapies e.g. beta-blockers or during a hypertensive crisis
Type of drug	PoM
Presentation	tablets, injection, powder for reconstitution
Dosage	*oral* – 25–50 mg b.d. *IV injection* – 5–10 mg over 20 minutes repeated after 20–30 minutes *IV infusion* – 200–300 micrograms/minute
Route of admin.	oral, IV injection or infusion
Contra-ind.	systemic lupus erythematosis (SLE), tachycardia
Side effects	nausea, postural hypotension, tachycardia, fluid retention, after prolonged or high dose therapy SLE-like syndrome
Interactions	*alcohol* – enhances hypotensive effect *anaesthetics* – enhances hypotensive effect *analgesics* – NSAIDs enhance hypotensive effect *antihypotensives* – enhance hypotensive effect *contraceptives* – combined oral contraceptives antagonize the hypotensive effect
Fetal risk	toxicity in animals therefore considered a teratogen, although there are no reported links to congenital defects in humans
Breastfeeding	considered safe

B.P.	**labetalol hydrochloride**
Proprietary	LABETALOL ®, TRANDATE ®
Group	antihypertensive – alpha and beta adrenoreceptor blocker
Uses/indications	hypertension in prenancy, hypertensive crisis
Type of drug	PoM
Presentation	tablets (orange), ampoules
Dosage	*oral* – 100 mg b.d. increased up to 800 mg in three to four evenly divided doses/day (max 2.4 g daily) *IV injection* – 50 mg over 1 minute repeated after 5 minutes (max. 200 mg) *IV infusion* – 20 mg/hr doubled after 30 minutes (max. 160 mg/hr)
Route of admin.	oral, IV injection or infusion
Contra-ind.	asthma, chronic obstructive airways disease, heart block
Side effects	postural hypotension, tiredness, weakness, epigastric pain, difficulty with micturition
Interactions	*alcohol* – enhances hypotensives effect *anaesthetics* – enhance hypotensive effect *analgesics* – NSAIDs enhance hypotensive effects *antacids* – cimetidine inhibits the metabolism and therefore increases the plasma concentration of labetalol *antidiabetics* – enhanced hypoglycaemic effects and masks warning signs such as tremor *antihistamines* – increased risk of ventricular arrythmia with terfenadine

Interactions	*anxiolytics and hypnotics* – enhance the hypotensive effect *corticosteroids* – antagonize the hypotensive effect *ergometrine* – increases peripheral vasoconstriction *contraceptives* – combined oral contraceptives antagonize the hypotensive effect
Fetal risk	caution in use – fetal growth deficiency, neonatal hypoglycaemia and bradycardia, the risk is greater in severe hypertension although these effects may be due to the disease itself and not the therapy
Breastfeeding	considered safe but monitor infant carefully

B.P.	methyldopa
Proprietary	METHYLDOPA ®, ALDOMET ®, DOPAMET®
Group	centrally acting antihypertensive
Uses/ indications	hypertension in pregnancy, hypertensive crisis where immediate effect is not necessary, can be used by asthmatics
Type of drug	PoM
Presentation	tablets, suspension, ampoules
Dosage	*oral* – 250 mg b.d. (t.d.s.) max. 3 g/day *IVI* – 250–500 mg repeated 6 hrly
Route of admin.	oral, IVI
Contra-ind.	history of depression, liver disease, phaeochromocytoma
Side effects	reduced if under 1 g/day, dry mouth, sedation, depression, fluid retention, haemolytic anaemia, SLE-like syndrome
Interactions	*alcohol* – enhances hypotensive effect *anaesthetics* – enhances hypotensive effect ++ *analgesics* – NSAIDs enhance hypotensive effect *antihypertensives* – potentiate hypotensive effect *anxiolytics and hypnotics* – enhance hypotensive effect *corticosteroids* – antagonize hypotensive effect *contraceptives* – antagonize hypotensive effect
Fetal risk	nil apparent but there are reports of teratogenicity in multiple therapy
Breastfeeding	amount secreted considered too small to be harmful

B.P.	nifedipine
Proprietary	ADALAT ®
Group	calcium channel blocker
Uses/indications	hypertensive crisis
Type of drug	PoM
Presentation	capsules (orange)
Dosage	10 mg stat
Route of admin.	oral preferably sublingual
Contra-ind.	continuous use in pregnancy
Side effects	headache, flushing, dizziness tachycardia and palpitatory may inhibit labour
Interactions	*antidiabetics* – may occasionally impair glucose intolerance *antiepileptics* – effect of nifedipine reduced by phenytoin and phenobarbitone *antihypertensives* – enhances the hypotensive effect
Fetal risk	toxicity in animals, hypotensive effect can reduce placental flow and cause decrease in fetal oxygenation
Breastfeeding	considered safe 3–4 hrs after dose

References

Briggs, G.G., Freeman, R.K., Yaffe, S.J. (1990). *Drugs In Pregnancy And Lactation: A Reference Guide To Fetal And Neonatal Risk.* 3rd edition. Baltimore: Williams and Wilkins.

British Medical Association and the Royal Pharmaceutical Society of Great Britain (1996). *British National Formulary.* No. 31, March, Avon: Bath Press.

Hopkins, S.J. (1995). *Drugs And Pharmacology For Nurses.* 12th edition. Edinburgh: Churchill Livingstone.

Kelly, S. (1993). 'Disorders caused by pregnancy'. In: Bennett, V.R., Brown, L.K. (Eds). *Myles Textbook For Midwives.* 12th edition. Chapter 20, pp. 310–317. Edinburgh: Churchill Livingstone.

Read, M.D., Golightly, P.W., Grant, E. (1996). *Drugs In Breast Milk.* 14th edition. Boehringer Ingelheim Ltd.

Further reading

Bennett, P. (1994). 'Pre-eclampsia I'. *Modern Midwife,* Vol. 4, No. 10, pp. 20–22.

Bennett, P. (1994). 'Pre-eclampsia IV'. *Modern Midwife,* Vol. 5(1), pp. 25–26.

Bellin, L. (1994). 'Aspirin and pre-eclampsia'. *British Medical Journal ,*Vol. 308, No. 6939, 14 May, pp. 1250–1251.

de Swiet, M. (1994). 'Pre-eclampsia III'. *Modern Midwife,* Vol. 4(12) pp. 20–22.

Duley, L. (1994). 'Maternal morbidity and eclampsia: the eclampsia trial'. *MIDIRS Midwifery Digest,* Vol. 4, No. 2, June, pp. 176–178.

Eclampsia Trial Collaboration Group (1995). 'Report on the trials findings'. *The Lancet,* Vol. 345, No 8963, 10th June, pp. 1455–1463.

Enkin, M., Kierse, M., Renfrew, M., Neisson, J. (1995). *A Guide To Effective Care In Pregnancy And Childbirth.* 2nd edition. Chapter 15, pp. 90–99. Oxford: Oxford University Press.

Findings of the CLASP trial (1994). *Lancet,* Vol 343, No. 8898, 12 March, pp. 619–629.

Massaud, M., Baldwin, S. (1994). 'Pre-eclampsia II'. *Modern Midwife,* Vol. 4 (11) pp. 21–22.

CHAPTER TEN

Antiseptics

These substances are also known as disinfectants, bacteriostats, bactericide and germicides. They will inhibit the growth of or kill micro-organisms. Antiseptics are usually applied to the body and disinfectants to equipment. Skin cleansers are also included in this chapter.

The student should be aware of:

•   the difference between antiseptics and antibiotics.

B.P.	chlorhexidine
Proprietary	HIBISCRUB ®, CHLORHEXIDINE ®, HIBISOL ®, HIBITANE ®
Group	antiseptic, – chlorhexidine salts, phenyl derivative
Uses/indications	skin preparation prior to surgery, cleansing of perineum and vulva, lubrication of the hands of the midwife
Type of drug	N/A
Presentation	prepared solutions
Dosage	N/A
Route of admin.	topical
Contra-ind.	avoid contact with the eyes, brain meninges and middle ear, not suitable before diathermy
Side effects	sensitivity
Interactions	N/A
Fetal risk	N/A
Breastfeeding	N/A

B.P.	povidine – iodine
Proprietary	BETADINE ®, SAVLON ® (powder)
Group	antiseptic – iodine compounds
Uses/indications	skin disinfection, pre and post operative, caution with diathermy
Type of drug	N/A
Presentation	prepared solutions, powders
Dosage	N/A
Route of admin.	topical
Contra-ind.	use on very low birth weight babies
Side effects	sensitivity
Interactions	N/A
Fetal risk	avoid use on very low birth weight babies
Breastfeeding	N/A

B.P.	surgical alcohol (isopropyl alcohol)
Proprietary	
Group	alcoholic cleanser
Uses/indications	preparation of the skin prior to injection
Type of drug	GSL
Presentation	liquid, injection swabs
Dosage	N/A
Route of admin.	topical
Contra-ind.	broken skin, patients with burns, prior to using diathermy
Side effects	
Interactions	N/A
Fetal risk	N/A
Breastfeeding	N/A

B.P.	sodium chloride
Proprietary	NORMASOL ®, STERIPOD ®, STERAC ®
Group	saline skin cleanser
Uses/indications	cleansing of skin and wounds
Type of drug	
Presentation	sterile solution in ampoules and sachets
Dosage	N/A
Route of admin.	topical
Contra-ind.	N/A
Side effects	N/A
Interactions	N/A
Fetal risk	N/A
Breastfeeding	N/A

B.P.	
Proprietary	SAVLON ®
Group	antiseptic – phenyl derivative
Uses/indications	general purpose antiseptic, disinfectant and detergent
Type of drug	GSL
Presentation	liquid – chlorhexidine 1.5%, cetrimide 15%
Dosage	as instructed
Route of admin.	topical
Contra-ind.	sensitivity
Side effects	contamination by pseudomonous auregenosa – store in screw top bottles as sterile solutions
Interactions	N/A
Fetal risk	N/A
Breastfeeding	N/A

References

British Medical Association and Royal Pharmaceutical Society of Great Britain (1996). *British National Formulary.* No. 31, March, Avon: Bath Press.

Hopkins, S.J. (1995). *Drugs And Pharmacology For Nurses.* 12th edition. Edinburgh: Churchill Livingstone.

Further reading

Enkin, M., Keirse, M., Renfrew, M., Neilsson, J. (1995). *A Guide To Effective Care In Pregnancy And Childbirth.* Chapter 47, pp. 364–371, Chapter 45, pp. 340–348. Oxford: Oxford University Press.

Watkinson, M., Dyas, A. (1992). 'Staph. Aureus still colonizes the untreated umbilicus'. *Journal Of Hospital Infection,* Vol. 21, No. 2, June pp. 131–136.

CHAPTER ELEVEN

Contraceptives

This is a general term to describe an agent used to prevent conception. Those mentioned in this chapter are hormonal therapies and not devices.

The student should be aware of:

- Clause 4 of the Midwifes' Activities – 'the midwife has an important task in health counselling and education... which extends to family planning (Midwife's Code of Practice, May 1994),

- the availability of contraception,

- the importance of family planning,

- the process of contraception with a view to usage of Schering PC4 ®,

- the appropriateness of the contraceptive prescribed and

- the importance of counselling – advice on bleeding, missed pills, diarrhoea and vomiting, antibiotic administration and cessation of oral contraception prior to surgery.

B.P.	combined oestrogen/progestogen oral contraceptive
Proprietary	various – FEMODENE ®, MICROGYNON ®, EUGYNON ® etc.
Group	contraceptive – hormonal
Uses/indications	contraception, menstrual symptoms
Type of drug	PoM
Presentation	tablets in packs for one month with days numbered
Dosage	usually one tablet/day but refer to pack for instructions
Route of admin.	oral
Contra-ind.	pregnancy, migraine, liver disease including cholestatic jaundice, breastfeeding. Caution – arterial disease, smoking, hypertension obesity, diabetes mellitus with retinopathy and nephropathy, ischaemic heart disease, varicosities, depression, inflammatory bowel disease. Stop prior to surgery
Side effects	nausea, vomiting, headache, breast tenderness, changes in body weight, libido changes, DVT, intracyclic bleeding, ammenorrhoea, decreased menstrual bleeding
Interactions	*antibiotics* – broad spectrum – reduce effect *anticoagulants* – antagonizes the effect of warfarin *antiepileptics* – phemobarbitone and phenytoin accelerate metabolism and reduce contraceptive effect *beta-blockers* – antagonize hypotensive effect

Fetal risk	evidence suggests no harmful effects to fetus although there is teratogenicity in animals (US studies have found a small risk of 0.07% of all pregnancies exposed to the oral contraceptive pill)
Breastfeeding	suppressed lactation, contraindicated until at least six weeks after birth

B.P.	progesterone only pill
Proprietary	MICRONOR ®, FEMULEN ®, MICROVAL ®, NORGESTON ®, NEOGEST ®, NORIDAY ®
Group	contraceptive – hormonal
Uses/indications	contraception, alternative to oestrogens – higher failure rate, suitable in smokers, hypertension, valvular heart disease, diabetes mellitus, migraine
Type of drug	PoM
Presentation	tablets in cyclical packs
Dosage	usually 1 tablet/day but refer to pack instructions – must be taken at the same time each day
Route of admin.	oral
Contra-ind.	pregnancy, undiagnosed vaginal bleeding, severe arterial disease
Side effects	menstrual irregularities, nausea, vomiting, menstrual symptoms, weight change, depression
Interactions	*antibiotics* – Rifamycins – increase metabolism and therefore reduce effect *anticoagulants* – antagonizes effect of warfarin *antidiabetics* – antagonizes the hypoglycaemic effects *antiepileptics* – reduce contraceptive effect
Fetal risk	high doses may be teratogenic in the first trimester (US studies have found a 0.07 % risk)
Breastfeeding	not contraindicated but not before three weeks postpartum

B.P.	medroxyprogesterone acetate
Proprietary	DEPOPROVERA ®
Group	parenteral progesterone only contraceptive
Uses/indications	interim or long term contraception – 12 weeks duration
Type of drug	PoM
Presentation	aqueous suspension in vials
Dosage	150 mg in first 5 days of menstrual cycle or within 5 days of parturition, repeat in 12 weeks
Route of admin.	IM
Contra-ind.	as for oral preparations
Side effects	all over rash, nausea, giddiness, heavy bleeding during menses or postpartum, delay in return of fertility, menstrual disturbances
Interactions	as for oral preparations
Fetal risk	as for oral preparations
Breastfeeding	withold first dose until 5–6 weeks postpartum – but preparation does not suppress lactation

B.P.	norethisterone enanthate
Proprietary	NORISTERAT ®
Group	parenteral progesterone only contraceptive
Uses/indications	short term or interim contraception, 8 weeks duration
Type of drug	PoM
Presentation	oily preparation in ampoules
Dosage	deep IM – 200 mg in first 5 days of cycle or immediately following parturition, repeat in 8 weeks
Route of admin.	deep IM
Contra-ind.	as for oral preparations
Side effects	
Interactions	as for oral preparations
Fetal risk	as for oral preparations
Breastfeeding	withold when neonates have severe jaundice requiring medical treatment

B.P.	levonorgestrel
Proprietary	NORPLANT ®
Group	parenteral progesterone only contraceptive
Uses/indications	contraception, duration 5 years
Type of drug	PoM
Presentation	capsules for implant
Dosage	6 implant capsules inserted in first 5 days of menstrual cycle, preferably 1st day or 21 days after parturition, precautions for 5 days after implant
Route of admin.	sub-dermal
Contra-ind.	as for oral preparations
Side effects	irregular prolonged bleeding, ammenorrhoea
Interactions	as for oral preparations
Fetal risk	as for oral preparations
Breastfeeding	as for oral preparations

B.P.	
Proprietary	SCHERING PC4 ®
Group	contraceptive – emergency
Uses/indications	emergency contraception within 3 days (72 hrs) of unprotected intercourse
Type of drug	PoM
Presentation	tablets
Dosage	2 tablets – levonorgestrel 250 µg, ethinyloestradiol 50 ug – repeat in 12 hrs
Route of admin.	oral
Contra-ind.	*pregnancy,* history of thrombosis, history of focal migraine, overdue menstrual bleeding or unprotected intercourse more than 72 hrs previously
Side effects	nausea, vomiting, headache, dizziness, breast discomfort, menstrual irregularities
Interactions	antibiotics – ampicillin and others may impair the action of this preparation
Fetal risk	*abortifacient* but pregnancy may continue, monitor for signs of ectopic pregnancy. In theory because there is no organogenesis at 72 hrs there should be no teratogenicity
Breastfeeding	safety has not been established and therefore this drug should not be administered during breastfeeding

References

Briggs, G.G., Freeman, R.K., Yaffe, S.J. (1990). *Drugs In Pregnancy And Lactation: A Reference Guide To Fetal And Neonatal Risk.* 3rd edition. Baltimore: Williams and Wilkins.

British Medical Association and the Royal Pharmaceutical Society of Great Britain (1996). *British National Formulary.* No. 31, March, Avon: Bath Press.

Hopkins, S.J. (1995). *Drugs And Pharmacology For Nurses.* 12th edition Edinburgh: Churchill Livingstone.

Read, M.D., Golightly, P.W., Grant, E. (1996). *Drugs In Breast Milk.* 14th edition. Boehringer Ingelheim Ltd

SCHERING ™ – data sheets – SCHERING PC4 ®, NORISTERAT ®

Further reading

Bennett, V.R., Brown, L.K. (1993). *Myles Textbook For Midwives.* 12th edition. Edinburgh: Churchill Livingstone (see in the index under Family planning and contraception).

Faculty of Family Planning of the Royal College of Obstetricians and Gynaecologists (1995). 'Guidelines on discussing pill risks'. *Family Planning Association,* London, 26 Oct.

Keller, S. (1995). 'When to begin postpartum methods'. *Network,* Vol. 15, No. 3, March, pp. 18–23.

O'Sullivan, S., O'Connor, R.A. (1994). 'Do hospital staff gave correct advice about the combined pill?'. *British Journal Of Family Planning,* Vol. 20, No. 1, April, pp. 6–7.

CHAPTER TWELVE

Antihistamines

Histamine is present in animal tissues and some release occurs after injury but also after an allergic reaction and gives rise to urticaria, asthma, hayfever and ultimately *anaphylaxis*.

Antihistamines are palliative agents because they neither destroy nor prevent the release of histamine but act by blocking access to histamine receptor sites and thereby inhibiting an allergic reaction.

The student should be aware of:

- the physiology related to allergic response,

- the most common factors causing allergic response treatment for anaphylactic shock and

- interactions of drug therapy which may produce an allergic response i.e. cimetidine.

B.P.	chlorpheniramine
Proprietary	PIRITON ®
Group	antihistamine – sedative
Uses/indications	urticaria, hayfever, allergic rhinitis, insect bites, drug allergies, ANAPHYLAXIS
Type of drug	PoM, GSL
Presentation	tablets (ivory), syrup, ampoules
Dosage	12–16 mg/day divided into 4 mg 6–8 hrly
Route of admin.	oral, IM, slow IV injection (see chapter on emergency drugs)
Contra-ind.	epilepsy, hepatic disease, asthma as it has little effect on allergic bronchospasm
Side effects	drowsiness, lassitude, dizziness, dry mouth, blurred vision, headache, gastro-intestinal disturbances
Interactions	*alcohol* – potentiates sedative action *antidepressants* – enhances sedative effect – anticholinergic effect intensified with MAOIs *antidiabetics* – depressed thrombocyte count *antiepileptics* – inhibits the metabolism of phenytoin *antihistamines* – concommitant therapy **not** recommended *anxiolytics and hypnotics* – enhance the sedative effect
Fetal risk	no evidence of teratogenicity but manufacturers advise avoidance, use in the 3rd trimester may result in reactions in the neonate
Breastfeeding	secreted in significant amounts with no known effects but avoidance advised, it may also inhibit lactation

B.P.	terfenadine
Proprietary	own brand, TRILUDAN ®, ALLEREZE ®, HISTAFEN ®, SELDANE ®, TERFENOR ®, TERFOX ®
Group	antihistamine – non sedative
Uses/indications	symptomatic relief of allergic hayfever, urticaria
Type of drug	P
Presentation	tablets (white – scored)
Dosage	120 mg daily (60 mg b.d.)
Route of admin.	oral
Contra-ind.	hepatic disease, epilepsy, allergic asthma, pre-existing ventricular arrythmias
Side effects	? hair loss, less drowsiness, syncope, allergic urticaria, ventricular arrythmias
Interactions	*antiarrythmics* – increased risk of ventricular arrythmia *antibiotics* – inhibited by erythromycin and other macrolides *antidepressants* – tricyclics increase ventricular arrythmias *antidiabetics* – as for chlorpheniramine *antihistamines* – concommitant therapy **not** recommended *anxiolytics and hypnotics* – enhanced sedative effect
Fetal risk	as for chlorpheniramine
Breastfeeding	as for chlorpheniramine

References

ALLEN AND HANBURY ™ – data sheets – PIRITON ®

Briggs, G.G., Freeman, R.K., Yaffe, S.J. (1990). *Drugs In Pregnancy And Lactation: A Reference Guide To Fetal And Neonatal Risk.* 3rd edition. Baltimore: Williams and Wilkins.

British Medical Association and the Royal Pharmaceutical Society of Great Britain (1996). *British National Formulary.* No. 31, March, Avon: Bath Press.

Hopkins, S.J. (1995). *Drugs And Pharmacology For Nurses.* 12th edition. Edinburgh: Churchill Livingstone.

CHAPTER THIRTEEN

Hypoglycaemics

These are agents which reduce the excessive level of glucose in the blood, which is a feature of diabetes.

Insulin is a fuel regulating hormone, which controls the amount of glucose in the blood. Diabetics have a deficiency of insulin and therefore have a raised blood glucose level. There are three groups available – rapid acting, intermediate acting and long acting.

Women who are either insulin-dependent diabetics or gestational diabetics should be cared for by a medical diabetic consultant as well as a consultant obstetrician.

This chapter discusses the treatment used during pregnancy and does not address oral hypoglycaemics, such as glibenclamide, as they are rarely used during pregnancy.

The student should be aware of:

*   the physiology and pathophysiology of diabetes,

*   the treatment of diabetes,

*   the methods for diagnosing 'gestational diabetes',

*   the sequelae of a diabetic pregnancy,

*   local protocols for the care and treatment for diabetic mothers during ante, intra and postpartum periods and

*   care of the neonate after diabetic pregnancy.

B.P.	soluble insulins
Proprietary	HUMAN ACTRAPID ®, HUMAN VELOSULIN ®, HUMULIN ®
Group	short acting insulin
Uses/ indications	insulin-dependant diabetes mellitus, diabetic ketoacidosis, insulin dependant gestational diabetes
Type of drug	PoM
Presentation	ampoules, pre-prepared cartridges
Dosage	according to agreed regimen and according to patient requirements
Route of admin.	sub-cutaneous, IM, IV injection/infusion
Contra-ind.	reduce dosage in renal impairment
Side effects	hypoglycaemia, local reactions, fat hypertrophy at injection sites
Interactions	*alcohol* – enhances the hypoglycaemic effect *beta-blockers* – enhances hypoglycaemic effect and masks the warning signs e.g. tremor *corticosteroids* – antagonize the hypoglycaemic effect *contraceptives* – antagonize the hypoglycaemic effect
Fetal risk	insulin is an antagonist to surfactant production, some evidence of fetal growth deficiency, frequent antenatal surveillance is recommended. If the diabetes is poorly controlled, US studies have reported a 2–4 times greater probability of congenital defects induced prior to 7 weeks gestation and are usually responsible for the higher rate of first trimester abortions amongst this client group
Breastfeeding	insulin is a natural constituent of blood and is not secreted in breast milk

B.P.	biphasic isophane insulin
Proprietary	MIXTARD 30/70 ®, HUMAN MIXTARD ® (various concentrations), HUMULIN ®
Group	intermediate acting insulins
Uses/indications	insulin-dependant diabetes mellitus, insulin-dependant gestational diabetes
Type of drug	PoM
Presentation	ampoules, pre-prepared cartridges
Dosage	according to agreed regimen and according to patient requirements
Route of admin.	sub-cutaneous
Contra-ind.	as for soluble insulin
Side effects	hypoglycaemia, protamine can cause an allergic reaction, fat hypertrophy at injection sites
Interactions	as for soluble insulin
Fetal risk	as for soluble insulin
Breastfeeding	as for soluble insulin

B.P.	insulin zinc suspension
Proprietary	HUMAN MONOTARD ®
Group	long acting insulin
Uses/indications	insulin-dependant diabetes mellitus, insulin-dependant gestational diabetes
Type of drug	PoM
Presentation	ampoules
Dosage	according to agreed regimen and patient requirements
Route of admin.	sub-cutaneous
Contra-ind.	as for soluble insulin
Side effects	as for soluble insulin
Interactions	as for soluble insulin
Fetal risk	as for soluble insulin
Breastfeeding	as for soluble insulin

Examples of insulin regimes
(subject to alteration according to individual patient requirements)

Short acting insulin
SUB-CUTANEOUS
- usually administered 15–30 minutes prior to meals
- effective after 30–60 minutes
- peak effect after 2–4 hours
- duration 8 hours.

N.B. human preparations have more rapid onset and shorter durations.

INTRAVENOUS
- half life is 5 minutes and no longer effective after 30 minutes.

Intermediate and long acting insulin
SUB-CUTANEOUS
- onset 1–2 hours
- peak effect 4–12 hours
- duration 16–35 hours.

Modified insulins, such as biphasic isophane insulin e.g. *Mixtard 30/ 70 ®* or insulin zinc e.g. *Human Monotard ®* mean that the insulin can be absorbed slower and act more smoothly. In pregnancy this is useful as dose adjustment may be required.

Insulin therapy is usually substituted for oral therapy in pregnancy and oral hypoglycaemics should not be used during breastfeeding.

References

Briggs, G.G., Freeman, R.K., Yaffe, S.J. (1990). *Drugs In Pregnancy and Lactation: A Reference Guide To Fetal And Neonatal Risk.* 3rd edition. Baltimore: Williams and Wilkins.

British Medical Association and the Royal Pharmaceutical Society of Great Britain (1996). *British National Formulary.* No 31, March, Avon: Bath Press.

Hopkins, S.J. (1995). *Drugs And Pharmacology For Nurses.* 12th edition. Edinburgh: Churchill Livingstone.

Read, M.D., Golightly, P.W., Grant, E. (1996). *Drugs In Breast Milk.* 14th edition. Boehringer Ingelheim Ltd

Further reading

Bennett, V.R., Brown, L.K. (1993). *Myles Textbook For Midwives.* 12th edition. Edinburgh: Churchill Livingstone (see in the index under Diabetes).

Enkin, M., Keirse, M., Renfrew, M., Neilsson, J. (1995). *A Guide To Effective Care In Pregnancy And Childbirth.* 2nd edition. Chapter 20, pp. 126–134. Oxford: Oxford University Press.

With thanks to Jackie Maslin RGN, RM in compiling this chapter.

CHAPTER FOURTEEN

Intravenous Fluids

These are solutions of electrolytes which may be used as carriers or as described to maintain the electrolyte balance of the body when intra or extra cellular water changes occur e.g. in haemorrhage, dehydration or ketoacidosis.

Plasma expanders are used when there is sudden acute blood or plasma loss leading to a fall in blood pressure and the remaining blood cells collapse to try to redress the balance.

Drugs should *not* be added to infusions of sodium bicarbonate, amino acids, mannitol, blood products or specially prepared fat emulsions such as are used in Neonatal Intensive Care Units for feeding neonates (total parenteral nutrition) via the intravenous route.

Instructions as to storage and degradation of solutions should be noted and any deviation either from instructions or within the solution should indicate stopping the infusion.

Additive labels should be used to indicate what has been added to the solution, time, strength and, if relevant, expiry time/date, as well as patient identity and the signature of the practitioners checking the infusion. The practitioner must also be aware of the suitability of the additive to the electrolyte solution and where to refer any enquiries.

Intravenous fluids (in common usage)
Sodium chloride 0.9%
Isotonic solution – used in fluid replacement and electrolyte balance as an IV infusion, as a carrier for injections in which the prescribed drug requires reconstitution, or as a 'flush' for IV cannulae.

Glucose 5%

Used as an intravenous infusion (IVI) for fluid replacement and balance, used where there is dehydration without severe electrolyte loss, also used when there is an insulin infusion for the prevention of diabetic ketoacidosis e.g. during diabetic labours.

Dextrose saline

Sodium chloride 0.18% + gluose 4% – used as IVI to replace fluid and to restore electrolyte balance.

Hartmanns solution

Isotonic solution – used as IVI to replace fluid and restore electrolyte balance, often used in obstetrics as a carrier for syntocinon infusions or for 'pre-loading' prior to, and during epidural analgesia.

Water for injection

Used to reconstitute drugs prescribed as IV injection.

Potassium chloride + glucose

Used in severe electrolyte depletion – should be used with caution as rapid infusions are toxic to the heart, exact regimen is to be specified by the prescriber.

Potassium chloride + sodium chloride

As above, specified by the prescriber.

Potassium chloride + glucose + sodium chloride

As above, specified by the prescriber.

Plasma expanders

HAEMACEL ®, GELOFUSINE ® – used when there is low blood volume and after an initial 500–1000 ml further doses are given depending on the patients condition.

References

British Medical Association and the Royal Pharmaceutical Society of Great Britain (1996). *British National Formulary.* No. 31, March, Avon: Bath Press.

Hopkins, S.J. (1995). *Drugs And Pharmacology For Nurses.* 12th edition. Edinburgh: Churchill Livingstone.

CHAPTER FIFTEEN

Immunoglobulins

These are antibodies, present in the blood, which by specific and direct action defend the body against invading bacteria or organisms. The Anti-D immunoglobulin is used in treatment of Rhesus iso-immunization in women whose blood is Rhesus negative. This immunoglobulin, given via injection, coats the fetal cells which may have leaked into the maternal circulation following a sensitizing episode and thus preventing the woman becoming Rhesus iso-immunized.

Some antibodies that are present in maternal blood require consultation with Regional Blood Transfusion Centres as to their relevance to the mother and to the fetus/neonate.

Other uses of immunoglobulins include those used as vaccines e.g. hepatitis, rabies and tetanus.

The student should be aware of:

- blood grouping and Rhesus evaluation,

- the aetiology of Rhesus iso-immunization,

- prevention of iso-immunization,

- what action should be taken when there is a possibility that iso-immunization could occur e.g. in antepartum haemorrhage,

- counselling to prevent iso-immunization,

- the sequlae to mother and fetus/neonate of Rhesus iso-immunization and

- an awareness of other antibodies present in blood e.g. Lewis, Kell, Duffy, anti E and Anti Fy etc.

B.P.	anti D (Rh) immunoglobulin
Proprietary	PARTBULIN ® (see manufacturers leaflet for dosage instructions)
Group	immunoglobulins – specific
Uses/indications	to prevent Rhesus iso-immunization
Type of drug	PoM
Presentation	pre-prepared vials
Dosage	after any potentially sensitizing episode e.g. vaginal bleeding of uterine origin, abortion or amniocentesis up to 20 weeks gestation – 250 units per episode (within 72 hrs). Following sensitizing episode after 20 weeks e.g. birth of Rhesus positive infant, antepartum haemorrhage – 500 units (within 72 hrs). Dosage may vary according to the titre of fetal cells detected
Route of admin.	IM
Contra-ind.	
Side effects	soreness at injection site
Interactions	N/A
Fetal risk	N/A
Breastfeeding	N/A

N.B. In some centres Anti D is administered prophylactically – 500 units at 28 weeks and 34 weeks gestation and immediately at delivery in women who are Rhesus negative.

When evaluating titres, the date of the last dose of Anti D should be included as the antibodies persist in circulation and may give a falsely high reading.

Rubella vaccine can also be administered in the postpartum period with Anti D, providing that separate syringes are used and they are administered in contralateral (opposite side) limbs. If blood transfusion was necessary, then rubella vaccination should delayed for three months.

MMR vaccine should *not* be given within three months of Anti D immunoglobulin.

References
British Medical Association and the Royal Pharmaceutical Society of Great Britain (1996). *British National Formulary.* No. 31, March, Avon: Bath Press.
Hopkins, S.J. (1995). *Drugs And Pharmacology For Nurses.* 12th edition. Edinburgh: Churchill Livingstone.

Further reading
Bennett, V.R., Brown, L.K. (1993). 'Jaundice and infection'. In: Bennett, V.R., Brown, L.K. (1993). *Myles Textbook For Midwives.* 12th edition. Chapter 34, pp. 543–548. Edinburgh: Churchill Livingstone.

CHAPTER SIXTEEN

Oxytocics

Oxytocics are drugs which are used to stimulate uterine contractions. Used in obstetrics to augment labour, expedite delivery of the fetus and, in the third stage, the delivery of the placenta and to halt postpartum haemorrhage.

The student should be aware of:

- the physiology of labour,

- reasons for prolonged, incoordinate labour/contractions,

- the physical, psychological and chemical factors which could diminish contractions,

- reasons to expedite delivery,

- research pertaining to managed and physiological third stage of labour,

- appropriate emergency action to be taken in the event of syntocinon overdose,

- the local emergency protocol for postpartum haemorrhage,

- the sequelae of oxytocin administration in mother and neonate,

- local protocols for the induction and augmentation of labour including contra-indications to therapy e.g. cord prolapse, cephalo-pelvic disproportion, malpresentation, placenta praevia, antepartum haemorrhage and cautions in pre-disposition to uterine rupture, multiple pregnancy, grande multiparity, polyhydramnios, previous caesarean section and

- the action of oxytocin, ergometrine and syntometrine.

B.P.	oxytocin
Proprietary	SYNTOCINON ®
Group	oxytocic
Uses/indications	augmentation/induction of labour, control of postpartum haemorrhage
Type of drug	PoM
Presentation	ampoules (5 units, 10 units)
Dosage	according to protocol
Route of admin.	IM, IVI or slow IV injection
Contra-ind	hypertonic uterine contractions, mechanical obstruction to delivery, fetal distress, where vaginal delivery is inadvisable, oxytocin resistant uterine inertia, severe pre-eclampsia, cardiovascular disease
Side effects	uterine spasm, uterine hyperstimulation, water intoxication, hypernatraemia, nausea, vomiting, rashes, ANAPHYLAXIS, placental abruption, amniotic fluid embolism – ARM or SRM should be diagnosed prior to beginning therapy
Interactions	*anaesthetics* – can potentiate the hypotensive effect and may cause arrythmias, the oxytocic effect may be reduced *prostaglandins* – uterotonic effect potentiated
Fetal risk	fetal distress, asphyxia, IUD, infusions in labour may be associated with neonatal jaundice
Breastfeeding	nil of note

B.P.	ergometrine maleate with syntocinon
Proprietary	SYNTOMETRINE ®
Group	oxytocic
Uses/Indications	to expedite placental delivery, to control haemorrhage
Type of drug	PoM
Presentation	ampoules
Dosage	1 ampoule – ergometrine 500 µg + 5 units oxytocin in 1 ml
Route of admin.	IM
Contra-ind.	pre-eclampsia, renal impairment, 1st and 2nd stages of labour, hepatic, cardiac or pulmonary disease, previous adverse reaction
Side effects	nausea, vomiting, headache, dizziness, tinnitus, chest pain, palpitations, vaso-constriction, myocardial infarction, pulmonary oedema, stroke, muscle pain
Interactions	
Fetal risk	ABORTIFACIENT
Breastfeeding	nil noted

B.P.	**ergometrine maleate**
Proprietary	ERGOMETRINE ®
Group	oxytocic-like substance
Uses/indications	postpartum haemorrhage (rarely used)
Type of drug	PoM
Presentation	ampoules, tablets
Dosage	*IM* – 200–500 µg *oral* – 0.5–1 mg *IV* – 125–250 µg (rarely used)
Route of admin.	IM, oral
Contra-ind.	pregnancy, 1st and 2nd stages of labour, as for syntometrine
Side effects	as for syntometrine
Interactions	
Fetal risk	ABORTIFACIENT
Breastfeeding	nil noted

References

Briggs, G.G., Freeman, R.K., Yaffe, S.J. (1990). *Drugs In Pregnancy And Lactation: A Reference Guide To Fetal And Neonatal Risk.* 3rd edition. Baltimore: Williams and Wilkins.

British Medical Association and the Royal Pharmaceutical Society of Great Britain (1996). *British National Formulary.* No. 31, March, Avon: Bath Press.

Hopkins, S.J. (1995). *Drugs And Pharmacology For Nurses.* 12th edition. Edinburgh: Churchill Livingstone.

Read, M.D., Golightly, P.W., Grant, E. (1996). *Drugs In Breast Milk. 14th* edition, Boehringer Ingelheim Ltd

Further reading

Enkin, M., Keirse, M., Renfrew, M., Neilsson, J. (1995). *A Guide To Effective Care In Pregnancy And Childbirth.* 2nd edition. Oxford: Oxford University – various references occur throughout the book including a section on the techniques of labour induction.

Sleep, J. (1993). 'Complications of the third stage of labour'. In: Bennett, V.R., Brown, L.K. (1993). *Myles Textbook For Midwives.* 12th edition. Chapter 29, pp.462–470. Edinburgh: Churchill Livingstone.

William, J. (1993). 'Prolonged pregnancy and disorders of uterine action'. In: Bennett, V.R., Brown, L.K. (Eds). *Myles Text Book For Midwives.* 12th edition. Chapter 25, pp. 393–401 Edinburgh: Churchill Livingstone.

CHAPTER SEVENTEEN

Prostaglandins

Prostaglandins are hormones secreted by various body tissues e.g. uterine and cardiac muscle, semen and the lungs.

In obstetrics, prostaglandins are used to ripen the uterine cervix and cause contractions during the induction of labour.

The students should be aware of:

* the indications for induction of labour,

* local protocols for induction of labour – specifically the dosage used,

* the action of the prostaglandins with respect to termination of pregnancy and the side effects and

* the use of the Bishops Score in induction of labour.

B.P.	dinoprostone
Proprietary	PROSTIN E2 ®
Group	prostaglandins
Uses/indications	induction of labour – ripening of the cervix for labour
Type of drug	PoM
Presentation	vaginal gel or pessaries (also tablets, IV solution, extra-amniotic solution but rarely used)
Dosage	refer to protocol. Usually 1–2 mg depending on parity, and Bishops Score – repeat 6 hrly
Route of admin.	oral, per vaginum (not intra-cervical)
Contra-ind.	previous sensitivity, cephalo-pelvic disproportion, ruptured membranes, previous caesarean section or uterine surgery, untreated pelvic infection, grande multiparity, fetal distress. Avoid in cervicitis or vaginitis
Side effects	nausea, vomiting, diarrhoea, severe uterine contractions, overdosage leading to uterine rupture
Interactions	*oxytocics* – uterotonic effect enhanced
Fetal risk	ABORTIFACIENT
Breastfeeding	not applicable

B.P.	gemeprost
Proprietary	CERVAGEM ®
Group	prostaglandin
Uses/indications	used in cervical ripening during therapeutic termination
Type of drug	PoM
Presentation	pessaries
Dosage	dependent on stage of pregnancy and indication
Route of admin.	per vaginum
Contra-ind.	chronic obstructive airways disease, cardiovascular insufficiency, raised intraocular pressure, cervicitis, vaginitis, caution should be used with previous uterine surgery
Side effects	vaginal bleeding, uterine pain, nausea, vomiting, diarrhoea, headache, flushing, chills, dizziness, muscle weakness, backache, dyspnoea, chest pain, mild pyrexia, uterine rupture especially with previous LSCS, grande multiparity
Interactions	oxytocics – enhances uterotonic effect
Fetal risk	ABORTIFACIENT
Breastfeeding	not applicable

References

British Medical Association and the Royal Pharmaceutical Society of Great Britain (1996). *British National Formulary*. No. 31, March, Avon: Bath Press.

Hopkins, S.J. (1995). *Drugs And Pharmacology For Nurses*. 12th edition. Edinburgh: Churchill Livingstone.

Further reading

Enkin, M., Keirse, M., Renfrew, M., Neilsson, J. (1995). *A Guide To Effective Care In Pregnancy And Childbirth*. 2nd edition. Oxford: Oxford University Press. Chapter 39 and Chapter 40, as well as various other references throughout this book.

Williams, J. (1993). 'Prolonged pregnancy and disorders of uterine action'. In: Bennett, V.R., Brown, L.K. (Eds). *Myles Textbook For Midwives*. Chapter 25, pp. 392–393, 12th edition. Edinburgh: Churchill Livingstone.

CHAPTER EIGHTEEN

Myometrial Relaxants

These drugs are sympathomimetics and relax uterine muscle, hopefully preventing premature labour. Mostly they are used to delay delivery until corticosteroid therapy is complete. Some are used as antagonists to oxytocin hyperstimulation of the uterus during induction or augmentation of labour.

Their use is indicated between 24–33 weeks gestation in uncomplicated cases.

The student should be aware of:

•   what constitutes premature labour,

•   local protocols for the management of premature labour and

•   the sequelae of the action of these drugs on the mother and fetus.

B.P.	ritodrine hydrochloride
Proprietary	YUTOPAR ®
Group	myometrial relaxant
Uses/indications	inhibition of uncomplicated premature labour between 24–33 weeks gestation, or to delay delivery by up to 48 hrs to administer glucocorticosteroids and implement other measures for neonatal well-being
Type of drug	PoM
Presentation	tablets (yellow), ampoules
Dosage	as per local protocols, in uterine hypertonicity — 50 micrograms/minute IV until the uterus relaxes
Route of admin.	oral, IM, IV (in 5% Dextrose)
Contra-ind.	if labour progresses after the maximum 350 microgram dose, cord compression, cardiac disease, pre-eclampsia, eclampsia, intra uterine infection, intra uterine death, obstetric haemorrhage, placenta praevia, 1st and 2nd trimester of pregnancy
Side effects	nausea, vomiting, sweating, tremor, tachycardia if over 140 bpm – cease infusion, palpitations, hypotension, increased tendency to uterine bleeding, pulmonary oedema, chest pain and tightness, use caution with hydration and if pulmonary oedema develops cease infusion
Interactions	*corticosteroids* – with a high dose of rotidrine and high dose of corticosteriods there is an increased risk of hypokalaemia

Interactions	loop diuretics and thiazides – risk of hypokalaemia *theophylline* – risk of hypokalaemia **Caution** – when IV in diabetic clients – glucose levels should be monitored and insulin regimes need adjusting accordingly
Fetal risk	increased risk of obstetric haemorrhage, intra uterine death, transient neonatal tachycardia
Breastfeeding	no data available

B.P.	salbutamol
Proprietary	VENTOLIN ®
Group	myometrial relaxant/bronchodilator
Uses/indications	inhibition of uncomplicated premature labour 24–33 weeks gestation, also used to antagonize hypertonic contractions
Type of drug	PoM
Presentation	ampoules, syrup, tablets, inhalers
Dosage	as per local protocols
Route of admin.	oral, IM, IV/infusion (in 5% Dextrose)
Contra-ind.	as for ritodrine – caution with diabetics
Side effects	fine tremor, tension, headache, peripheral vasodilation, tachycardia if over 140 bpm – cease infusion, hypersensitivity, pulmonary oedema – observe the volume of fluid infused
Interactions	as for ritodrine
Fetal risk	as for ritodrine
Breastfeeding	evidence for the safety of salbutamol during lactation – not conclusive

B.P.	terbutaline
Proprietary	BRICANYL ®, MONVENT ®
Group	myometrial relaxant/bronchodilator
Uses/indications	inhibition of uncomplicated labour 24–33 weeks gestation
Type of drug	PoM
Presentation	ampoules, syrup, tablets, inhalers
Dosage	as per local protocols
Route of admin.	IVI, sub-cutaneous, oral
Contra-ind.	as for ritodrine
Side effects	as for salbutamol
Interactions	as for ritodrine
Fetal risk	as for ritodrine
Breastfeeding	secreted in breastmilk but amounts are too small to be harmful

References

ALLEN AND HANBURYS ™ – data sheets – VENTOLIN ®

ASTRA ™ – data sheets – BRICANYL ®

Briggs, G.G., Freeman, R.K., Yaffe, S.J. (1990). *Drugs In Pregnancy And Lactation: A Reference Guide To Fetal And Neonatal Risk.* 3rd edition. Baltimore: Williams and Wilkins.

British Medical Association and the Royal Pharmaceutical Society of Great Britain (1996). *British National Formulary.* No. 31, March, Avon: Bath Press.

DUPHAR ™ – data sheets – YUTOPAR ®

Hopkins, S.J. (1995). *Drugs And Pharmacology For Nurses.* 12th edition. Edinburgh: Churchill Livingstone.

Read, M.D., Golightly, P.W., Grant, E. (1996). *Drugs In Breast Milk.* 14th edition. Boehringer Ingelheim Ltd.

CHAPTER NINETEEN

Rectal Preparations

Laxatives

These are medicines which loosen the bowel content and encourage evacuation. They are also known as aperients.

Haemorrhoid preparations

These come in the form of suppositories or topical creams and they contain local anaesthetics or corticosteroids.

The student should be aware of:

• the effect of progesterone on the alimentary tract musculature,

• factors predisposing to haemorrhoids and

• use of dietary measures to alleviate constipation.

B.P.	bisacodyl
Proprietary	DULCOLAX ®
Group	stimulant laxative
Uses/indications	constipation
Type of drug	GSL
Presentation	tablets (white), suppositories
Dosage	5–10 mg nocte, action over 10–12 hrs
Route of admin.	oral, p.r.
Contra-ind.	avoid in children
Side effects	abdominal cramps, not for prolonged use as it can cause atonic non-functioning colon and hypokalaemia
Interactions	no data available
Fetal risk	no data available
Breastfeeding	considered safe

B.P.	**docusate sodium**
Proprietary	NORGALAX MICRO-ENEMA ®
Group	stimulant laxative
Uses/indications	constipation
Type of drug	PoM
Presentation	enema
Dosage	120 mg in 10 g – single dose disposable pack
Route of admin.	p.r.
Contra-ind.	haemorrhoids, anal fissure
Side effects	local irritant
Interactions	N/A
Fetal risk	N/A
Breastfeeding	not secreted in breastmilk

B.P.	glycerol
Proprietary	
Group	stimulant laxative – rectal stimulant only
Uses/indications	constipation
Type of drug	GSL
Presentation	suppositories
Dosage	adult – 4 g = 1 suppository
Route of admin.	p.r.
Contra-ind.	anal fissure, haemorrhoids
Side effects	local irritation
Interactions	N/A
Fetal risk	N/A
Breastfeeding	N/A

B.P.	senna
Proprietary	SENOKOT ®
Group	stimulant laxatives
Uses/indications	constipation
Type of drug	GSL
Presentation	tablets (green/brown), granules (brown), syrup (brown)
Dosage	1–2 tablets nocte, granules 5–10 ml nocte, syrup 10–20 ml nocte
Route of admin.	oral
Contra-ind.	avoid abuse as it can cause atonic non-functioning colon and hypokalaemia
Side effects	abdominal cramps, local irritation
Interactions	no data available
Fetal risk	no reports of fetal or animal toxicity
Breastfeeding	standardized forms are considered safe

B.P.	lactulose
Proprietary	DUPHALAC ®
Group	osmotic laxative
Uses/indications	constipation
Type of drug	GSL
Presentation	solution, white crystalline powder
Dosage	15 ml b.d. (50% solution)
Route of admin.	oral
Contra-ind.	galactosaemia, intestinal obstruction
Side effects	flatulence, abdominal cramps and discomfort
Interactions	no data available
Fetal risk	no reports of teratogenicity or hazard to the fetus
Breastfeeding	no data available

Haemorrhoid preparations

Haemorrhoid preparations are combinations of ingredients such as soothing compounds e.g. local anaesthetic, and corticosteroids, e.g. hydrocortisone to alleviate the local inflammatory response. They may also contain mild astrigents, vasoconstrictors and heparinoids to help relieve the haemorrhoid.

Anusol ®

Cream, ointment, suppositories – applied twice daily after a bowel movement or one suppository twice a day – use neither for longer than seven days.

Scheriproct ®

Ointment or suppositories – apply twice a day for five to seven days (three to four times a day on first day if necessary), then once daily for a few days until symptoms have cleared, or one suppository daily after bowel movement for five to seven days.

Proctosedyl ®

Ointment or suppositories – apply twice daily after bowel movement or insert one suppository twice a day after bowel movement – do not use either for longer than seven days.

References

Briggs, G.G., Freeman, R.K., Yaffe, S.J. (1990). *Drugs In Pregnancy And Lactation: A Reference Guide To Fetal And Neonatal Risk.* 3rd edition. Baltimore: Williams and WIlkins.

British Medical Association and the Royal Pharmaceutical Society of Great Britain (1996). *British National Formulary.* No. 31, March, Avon: Bath Press.

Hopkins, S.J. (1995). *Drugs And Pharmacology For Nurses.* 12th edition. Edinburgh: Churchill Livingstone.

Read, M.D., Golightly, P.W., Grant, E. (1996). *Drugs In Breast Milk.* 14th edition. Boehringer Ingelheim Ltd

SOLVAY HEALTHCARE ™ – data sheets – LACTULOSE ®

CHAPTER TWENTY

Vaccines

A vaccine is a suspension of dead or disabled organisms which, when injested or injected, prevent, lessen or treat infections or disease. The most common vaccines used in midwifery are rubella and varicella.

The student should be aware of:

•   detection of low levels of rubella antibodies in a client,

•   when it is appropriate to give vaccines in the postnatal period,

•   the sequlae of either vaccination or of disease and

•   the possible side effects of vaccination.

B.P.	rubella vaccine
Proprietary	ALMEVAX ®, EREVAX ®
Group	vaccine – live
Uses/indications	vaccination where there are low levels of rubella antibodies or none detected
Type of drug	PoM
Presentation	ampoules
Dosage	0.5 ml deep sub-cutaneous/IM
Route of admin.	deep sub-cutaneous, IM
Contra-ind.	pregnancy or the intention to become pregnant within one month
Side effects	a mild form of the disease
Interactions	no data available
Fetal risk	theoretical risk of teratogenicity and therefore should be avoided unless the need for vaccination outweighs the risk to the fetus
Breastfeeding	available data suggests that breastfeeding is safe

B.P.	varicella zoster immunoglobulin
Proprietary	
Group	vaccine – immunoglobulin
Uses/indications	vaccination in women at risk of exposure
Type of drug	PoM
Presentation	ampoules
Dosage	1g IM within 10 days of exposure, repeated in three weeks if further exposed
Route of admin.	IM
Contra-ind.	
Side effects	
Interactions	
Fetal risk	
Breastfeeding	available data suggests that breastfeeding is safe

References

Briggs, G.G., Freeman, R.K., Yaffe, S.J. (1990). *Drugs In Pregnancy And Lactation: A Reference Guide To Fetal And Neonatal Risk.* 3rd edition. Baltimore: Williams and Wilkins.

British Medical Association and the Royal Pharmaceutical Society of Great Britain (1996). *British National Formulary.* No. 31, March, Avon: Bath Press.

Hopkins, S.J. (1995). *Drugs And Pharmacology For Nurses.* 12th edition. Edinburgh: Churchill Livingstone.

Read, M.D., Golightly, P.W., Grant, E. (1996). *Drugs In Breast Milk.* 14th edition, Boehringher Ingelheim Ltd.

CHAPTER TWENTY-ONE

Vitamins and Iron Preparations

Vitamins are factors in food necessary for growth and reproduction of living tissues. Some vitamins are fat soluble and others are water soluble.

Those of interest to the midwife are vitamins C, B_{12}, K and folic acid and are usually present in the diet. Supplements of vitamins C and K are rare but B_{12} and folic acid supplements are increasing.

Other elements present in food are minerals.

The student should be aware of:

- the importance of good nutrition in women of child-bearing age,

- what is considered malnutrition by the World Health Organization (WHO),

- the prevalence of malnutrition in local populations,

- the sequelae to mother and fetus of malnutrition and

- the foods which are part of a well-balanced healthy diet.

B.P.	vitamin B_{12} hydroxocobalamin
Proprietary	COBALIN-H ®, NEO-CYTAMEN ®
Group	vitamins - B complex
Uses/indications	*very rare in pregnancy,* pernicious anaemia, B_{12} deficiency
Type of drug	PoM
Presentation	ampoules
Dosage	1 mg repeat 5 times at 2–3 day intervals, maintainence dose 1 mg every 3 months
Route of admin.	deep IM
Contra-ind.	diagnosis of deficiency should be fully established
Side effects	
Interactions	
Fetal risk	maternal B_{12} deficiency results in poor fetal outcome – there are no reports of high maternal dosage at *term* and maternal or fetal complications
Breastfeeding	lack of B_{12} in the maternal diet can cause neonatal anaemia. Dietary supplements are recommended where deficiency is diagnosed

B.P.	folic acid
Proprietary	PRECONCEIVE ®
Group	vitamins - B complex
Uses/indications	prevention of neural tube defects, folate deficient megaloblastic anaemia
Type of drug	PoM, GSL (doses must not exceed 500 ug/day)
Presentation	tablets, syrup
Dosage	400 µg daily pre-conception or for the first 12 weeks of gestation in anaemia – 5 mg/day for 4 months
Route of admin.	oral
Contra-ind.	no data available
Side effects	no data available
Interactions	*antiepileptics* – folic acid has been known to reduce the phenytoin plasma concentration, therefore advice should be taken on supplementation
Fetal risk	no data available on overdosage
Breastfeeding	considered safe

Iron preparations

Iron (Fe) is a metallic element and a constituent of the haemoglobin molecule which is necessary to carry oxygen around the body via the blood.

Involved in iron absorption is vitamin C and to a lesser extent, folic acid. In theory, haemoglobin (Hb) concentration in the blood should rise 2g/100ml or 20g/l over 3–4 weeks of supplementation.

The student should be aware of:

- the WHO guidelines for diagnosis of anaemia,

- the aetiology and predisposing factors to anaemia,

- the physiology and pathophysiology of anaemia in pregnancy,

- the appropriateness and effectiveness of iron preparations in both anaemia and routinely in pregnancy,

- the different kinds of anaemia and their prognosis,

- the dietary sources of iron, Vitamin C and folic acid and

- the sequelae of anaemia in ante, intra and postnatal periods.

B.P.	ferrous sulphate
Proprietary	FEOSPAN ®, FERROGRAD ®
Group	iron salts
Uses/indications	iron deficiency anaemia
Type of drug	PoM
Presentation	tablets (white coated)
Dosage	1 tablet 200 mg/daily in prophylaxis or mild anaemia 2–3 tablets 400–600 mg/daily in therapeutic doses
Route of admin.	oral
Contra-ind.	diverticulitis, inflammatory bowel disease, anaemias other than iron deficiency
Side effects	nausea, gastric irritation, epigastric pain, diarrheoa or constipation, iron overload, darkening of the stools
Interactions	*antacids* – magnesium trisilicate reduces the absorbtion of iron
Fetal risk	no data available
Breastfeeding	considered safe

B.P.	Fe sorbitol compound
Proprietary	JECTOFER ®
Group	iron salts
Uses/indications	failure of oral therapy e.g. severe continuous blood loss, malabsorbtion
Type of drug	PoM
Presentation	ampoules
Dosage	calculated according to client weight and iron deficiency
Route of admin.	deep IM
Contra-ind.	liver and kidney disease (pyelonephritis), untreated UTI, early pregnancy, pre-existing cardiac anomalies
Side effects	pain at injection site, nausea, vomiting, dizziness, flushing, severe arrythmias, theoretical risk of myocardial infarction, urine may turn black
Interactions	
Fetal risk	
Breastfeeding	

N.B. Due to the risk of myocardial infarction, iron injections should be carried out under strict medical supervision. Defibrillation facilities and adrenaline must be immediately available.

It is also recommended that the course of oral iron should be stopped 48 hours prior to the IM course.

Other iron compounds

Fefol ®

Ferrous sulphate 150 mg and folic acid 500 µg – capsules (clear/green with brown, yellow and white pellets) – one capsule daily.

Pregaday ®

Ferrous fumarate (100 mg Fe) and folic acid (350 µg) tablets (brown) – one tablet daily.

References

Briggs, G.G., Freeman, R.K., Yaffe, S.J. (1990). *Drugs In Pregnancy And Lactation: A Reference Guide To Fetal And Neonatal Risk.* 3rd edition. Baltimore: Williams and Wilkins.

British Medical Association and the Royal Pharmaceutical Society of Great Britain (1996). *British National Formulary.* No. 31, March, Avon: Bath Press.

EVANS ™ – data sheets – FEFOL SPANSULES ®

Hopkins, S.J. (1992). *Drugs And Pharmacology For Nurses.* 12th edition. Edinburgh: Churchill Livingstone.

Read, M.D., Golightly, P.W., Grant, E. (1996). *Drugs In Breast Milk.* 14th edition. Boehringer Ingelheim Ltd.

Further reading

Enkin, M., Kierse, M., Renfrew, M., Neilsson. J. (1995). *A Guide To Effective Care On Pregnancy And Childbirth.* 2nd edition. Oxford: Oxford University Press. Chapter 6

LLoyd, C., Lewis, V. (1993). 'Diseases associated with pregnancy'. In: Bennett, V.R., Brown, L.K. (Eds). *Myles Textbook For Midwives.* 12th edition. Edinburgh: Churchill LIvingstone.

Montgomery, E. (1993). 'Iron and vitamin supplementation during pregnancy'. In: Alexander, J., Levy, V., Roch, S. (Eds). *Midwifery Practice - A Research Based Approach.* Basingstoke: Macmillan Press Ltd.

CHAPTER TWENTY-TWO

Anxiolytics and Hypnotics

These are used to lessen tension and excitement and to induce sleep. They may be prescribed for anxious clients or those unable to sleep in the antenatal period during hospitalization.

The student should be aware of:

- the effects tension has in exacerbating certain conditions and

- the addictive qualities of such preparations.

B.P.	temazepam
Proprietary	NORMISON ®
Group	hypnotic – benzodiazepine
Uses/indications	insomnia (short-term use)
Type of drug	PoM
Presentation	tablets (white)
Dosage	10–20 mg nocte
Route of admin.	oral
Contra-ind.	any history of drug/alcohol abuse, respiratory disease, myasthenia gravis, marked personality disorders
Side effects	drowsiness, light headedness
Interactions	*alcohol, analgesics, anaesthetics, antihistamines, antihypertensives –* all enhance the sedatory effect *antihistamines –* concommitant administration with diphenhydramine can cause intra uterine death or early neonatal death
Fetal risk	drowsiness, with large doses hypotonia, depression of neonatal respiration and withdrawal symptoms
Breastfeeding	avoid repeated doses – can lead to lethargy and weight loss in the infant – otherwise safe

References

Briggs, G.G., Freeman, R.K., Yaffe, S.J. (1990). *Drugs In Pregnancy And Lactation: A Reference Guide To Fetal And Neonatal Risk.* 3rd edition. Baltimore: Williams and Wilkins.

British Medical Association and the Royal Pharmaceutical Society of Great Britain (1996). *British National Formulary.* No. 31, March, Avon: Bath Press.

Hopkins, S.J. (1995). *Drugs And Pharmacology For Nurses.* 12th edition. Edinburgh: Churchill Livingstone.

Read, M.D., Golightly, P.W., Grant, E. (1996). *Drugs In Breast Milk.* 14th edition. Boehringer Ingelheim Ltd.

WYETH™ – data sheets – NORMISON ®

CHAPTER TWENTY-THREE

Antifungals

These are drugs used to combat fungal infections. They can be ingested or applied topically depending on the infection.

The student should be aware of:

- common antifungal infections in pregnancy,

- the physiology and pathophysiology which allows these infections to flourish and

- the appropriateness of the antifungal treatment prescribed.

B.P.	**nystatin**
Proprietary	NYSTAN ®
Group	antifungal
Uses/indications	candidasis
Type of drug	PoM
Presentation	oral suspension (yellow), tablets, pessaries, pastilles
Dosage	*oral* – 100 000 units q.d.s. for 7 days i.e. 1 pastille or 1 ml of suspension *p.v.* – 1–2 pessaries for 12–14 nights
Route of admin.	oral, per vaginum
Contra-ind.	
Side effects	nausea, vomiting, hypersensitivity
Interactions	no data available
Fetal risk	no reports of complications after administration in pregnancy
Breastfeeding	not secreted in breastmilk

B.P.	clotrimazole
Proprietary	CANESTAN ®
Group	antifungal
Uses/indications	candidasis
Type of drug	PoM, P
Presentation	cream (topical), pessaries
Dosage	see manufacturers instructions
Route of admin.	oral, p.v.
Contra-ind.	
Side effects	occasional local irritation
Interactions	*contraceptives* – may affect latex condoms and diaphragms
Fetal risk	use with caution as US studies show that when 1st trimester vaginitis was treated with this preparation had a small association with birth defects
Breastfeeding	no data available

References

Briggs, G.G., Freeman, R.K., Yaffe, S.J. (1990). *Drugs In Pregnancy And Lactation: A Reference Guide To Fetal And Neonatal Risk.* 3rd edition. Baltimore: Williams and Wilkins.

British Medical Association and the Royal Pharmaceutical Society (1996). *British National Formulary.* No. 31, March, Avon: Bath Press.

Hopkins, S.J. (1995). *Drugs And Pharmacology For Nurses.* 12th edition. Edinburgh: Churchill Livingstone.

Read, M.D., Golightly, P.W., Grant, E. (1996). *Drugs In Breast Milk.* 14th edition. Boehringer Ingelheim Ltd.

CHAPTER TWENTY-FOUR

Miscellaneous

This chapter contains the drugs which are used in midwifery that do not come under any previous title. These include some alternative medicines, as well as pharmaceutical preparations.

Any preparation should be prescribed by a recognized and registered practitioner in alternative therapy, just as with conventional medicine one would seek the advice of a doctor or pharmacist prior to taking a medicine.

The student is urged to examine Rule 41, further expanded in the Midwives Code of Practice (1994) and the more recent Guidelines for Professional Practice (1996) for guidance when a client is using or wishes to use alternative therapies.

Name	hamamelis virginica aka *witch hazel*
Uses/indications	varicosities, perineal trauma, herpes lesions
Type of drug	herbal remedy
Presentation	liquid
Dosage	as directed by practitioner
Route of admin.	topical
Contra-ind.	
Side effects	
Interactions	
Fetal risk	
Breastfeeding	

Name	marigold aka *calendula officinalis*
Uses/indications	perineal trauma, sore nipples, cystitis, thrush, herpes, nappy rash
Type of drug	herbal remedy
Presentation	ointment, infusion
Dosage	as directed by practitioner
Route of admin.	oral or topical
Contra-ind.	
Side effects	
Interactions	
Fetal risk	
Breastfeeding	

Name	arnica montana aka *leopards bane*
Uses/indications	first aid remedy in bruising and soreness e.g. episiotomy or other perineal trauma
Type of drug	homeopathic remedy
Presentation	tablet or suspension, cream
Dosage	as directed by homeopathic practitioner
Route of admin.	oral or topical
Contra-ind.	
Side effects	
Interactions	
Fetal risk	
Breastfeeding	

B.P.	peppermint water
Uses/indications	to ease colic/flatulence, and abdominal cramps
Type of drug	herbal remedy and is also used in aromatherapy
Presentation	*herbal tea* – to treat anaemia and mood swings *herbal suspension/infusion* – as indicated above *essential oil* – to treat nausea and vomiting
Dosage	as directed by practitioner
Route of admin.	oral, inhaled
Contra-ind.	
Side effects	
Interactions	
Fetal risk	
Breastfeeding	

B.P.	chlomiphene citrate
Proprietary	CLOMID ®, SERPHENE ®
Group	anti-oestrogen
Uses/indications	anovulatory infertility
Type of drug	PoM
Presentation	tablets
Dosage	50 mg/day for 5 days after the onset of menstruation – use for a *maximum* 3 cycles and under the supervision of a specialist centre
Route of admin.	oral
Contra-ind.	*pregnancy*, hepatic disease, abnormal uterine bleeding
Side effects	hot flushes, abdominal discomfort, withdraw if there are visual disturbances or ovarian hyperstimulation
Interactions	
Fetal risk	ectopic pregnancy, risk of multiple pregnancy, multiple effects on fetal development reported therefore pregnancy should be excluded before the next course is commenced
Breastfeeding	not applicable

B.P.	dexamethasone
Proprietary	ORADEXON ®, DECADRON ®
Group	corticosteroid
Uses/indications	to promote surfactant production in a fetus under 34 weeks gestation and where labour is imminent
Type of drug	PoM
Presentation	tablets, IM injection
Dosage	IM – 12 mg 12 hrly repeated after 7 days
Route of admin.	oral, IM
Contra-ind.	
Side effects	
Interactions	*analgesics* – increases the risk of gastro-intestinal bleed with aspirin and other NSAIDs *antidiabetics* – antagonizes the hypoglycaemic effects *antiepileptics* – phenobarbitone and phenytoin accelerate the metabolism of corticosteroids *antihypertensives* – antagonize the antihypertensive effect
Fetal risk	overdosage can effect the adrenal development of the fetus and neonate, however the benefits vastly outweigh the risks of administration
Breastfeeding	no data available

B.P.	**thyroxine**
Proprietary	ELTROXIN ®
Group	thyroid hormone
Uses/indications	hypothyroidism
Type of drug	PoM
Presentation	tablets
Dosage	as indicated by laboratory monitoring and the physician
Route of admin.	oral
Contra-ind.	thyrotoxicosis
Side effects	these usually occur with overdose – tachycardisa, palpitations, muscle cramps and other indications of an increased metabolic rate
Interactions	*anticoagulants* – the effect of warfarin is enhanced *antiepileptics* – phenobarbitone and phenytoin accelerate the metabolism of thyroxine
Fetal risk	monitor serum levels closely
Breastfeeding	maternal dosage may interfere with neonatal screening for hypothyroidism

B.P.	loperamide
Proprietary	IMODIUM ®
Group	anti-diarrhoeal
Uses/indications	acute/chronic diarrhoea
Type of drug	GSL
Presentation	capsules, syrup
Dosage	adjusted according to response
Route of admin.	oral
Contra-ind.	abdominal distension, acute ulcerative colitis
Side effects	abdominal cramps, urticaria
Interactions	no data available
Fetal risk	no reports linking loperamide with either human or animal toxicity found
Breastfeeding	one report in Australia recommends avoidance but otherwise no data is available

B.P.	aciclovir (acyclovir)
Proprietary	ZOVIRAX ®
Group	antiviral
Uses/indications	treatment of varicella zoster in pregnancy
Type of drug	PoM
Presentation	powder for reconstitution
Dosage	5 mg/kg t.d.s. by IV infusion over 1 hr
Route of admin.	IV infusion
Contra-ind.	renal impairment
Side effects	multiple including, rash, gastro-intestinal disturbances, on IV infusion – local inflammation
Interactions	
Fetal risk	use only when the benefits outweigh the risks as the number of exposures to the drug is too limited to assess the long term prognosis
Breastfeeding	significant amount secreted into breastmilk oral 5 day course – considered safe *IV* – insufficient information to allow classification as safe

B.P.	zidovudine (AZT)
Proprietary	RETROVIR ®
Group	antiviral
Uses/indications	management of HIV, possibly in the prevention of maternal-fetal HIV transmission
Type of drug	PoM
Presentation	capsules (white/blue band and blue, white/dark blue band) syrup, powder for reconstitution
Dosage	prevention of maternal/fetal transmission – over 14 weeks gestation oral – 100 mg 5 times a day until labour and delivery – *IVI* – 2mg/kg over 1 hr them 1 mg/kg/hr until the cord is clamped. If LSCS planned then commence the regime 4 hrs prior to delivery
Route of admin.	oral, IV infusion
Contra-ind.	low haemoglobin or neutrophil counts
Side effects	multiple, including gastro-intestinal disturbances, headache, rash, fever, anaemia
Interactions	*analgesics* – methadone increase the plasma concentrations of this drug *antiepileptics* – plasma phenytoin concentrations can increase or decrease
Fetal risk	use only if clearly indicated
Breastfeeding	not recommended

References

British Medical Association and the Royal Pharmaceutical Society of Great Britain (1996). *British National Formulary.* No. 31, March, Avon: Bath Press.

Hopkins, S.J. (1995). *Drugs And Pharmacology For Nurses.* 12th edition. Edinburgh: Churchill Livingstone.

Tiran, D., Mack, S. (1995). *Complementary Therapies For Pregnancy And Childbirth.* London: Balliere Tindall.

UKCC (1994). *The Midwives Code of Practice.* London: UKCC.

UKCC (1996). *Guidelines for Professional Practice* London: UKCC.

WELLCOME ™ – data sheets – ZOVIRAX ®

Further reading

Shepherd, C.M. (1994). *HIV Infection in Pregnancy.* Hale, Cheshire: Books for Midwives Press.

CHAPTER TWENTY-FIVE

Emergency Drugs

This chapter includes some of the drugs used in emergencies, such as eclampsia and haemorrhage. Also included is a list of drugs used in cardiac arrest or during treatment of anaphylactic shock.

These drugs are administered directly under the supervision of an expert e.g. a consultant anaesthetist and therefore the dosages are not included, unless they are particularly relevant.

Each student should quickly become familiar with the local protocols and policies which cover such emergencies and seek adequate training in resuscitation techniques.

B.P.	cimetidine
Proprietary	DYSPAMET ®, TAGAMET ®
Group	antacid
Uses/indications	labour where there is a high probability of LSCS, prior to emergency LSCS
Type of drug	PoM
Presentation	tablets (green), prepared ampoules for IV administration
Dosage	*oral* – 400 mg 8 hrly *IV injection* – slowly over 12 minutes – 200 mg
Route of admin.	oral, IV
Contra-ind.	see chapter 1
Side effects	see chapter 1
Interactions	see chapter 1
Fetal risk	see chapter 1
Breastfeeding	see chapter 1

B.P.	sodium citrate
Proprietary	
Group	antacid
Uses/indications	to reduce the acidity of gastric contents
Type of drug	PoM
Presentation	solution
Dosage	30 ml immediately prior to the induction of anaesthesia
Route of admin.	oral
Contra-ind.	
Side effects	
Interactions	
Fetal risk	
Breastfeeding	

Drugs used in the treatment of severe pre-eclampsia and eclampsia

B.P.	magnesium sulphate
Proprietary	
Group	anticonvulsant – muscle relaxant
Uses/indications	in pre-eclampsia and eclampsia
Type of drug	PoM
Presentation	ampoules
Dosage	according to local protocol
Route of admin.	IV infusion
Contra-ind.	
Side effects	*overdose* – loss of pastellar reflexes, weakness, nausea, sensation of warmth, flushing, drowsiness, slurred speech, double vision
Interactions	caution with aminoglycoside antibiotics within the first 24–48 hrs of birth
Fetal risk	fetal heart should be continuously monitored, neurological depression of the neonate includes respiratory depression, muscle weakness and loss of reflexes
Breastfeeding	secreted but considered safe
Antagonist	Calcium gluconate

N.B. According to the BNF, ECG monitoring is required during administration as well as blood pressure and signs of overdose.

B.P.	diazepam
Proprietary	VALIUM ®, DIAZEMULS ®
Group	benzodiazepine – sedative, hypnotic, muscle relaxant
Uses/indications	short term anxiety/insomnia, status epilepticus, eclampsia
Type of drug	PoM
Presentation	tablets, solution, emulsion, suppositories
Dosage	*oral* – anxiety – 2 mg t.d.s. increasing to 5–30 mg daily, else refer to protocols *suppositories* – rectal solution 5–15 mg slow *IV* – 5–10 mg repeated not less than 4 hrly
Route of admin.	oral, IM, IV, p.r.
Contra-ind.	history of drug or alcohol dependence, existing respiratory depression, mental illness including psychosis and phobia, *pregnancy* and *breastfeeding*
Side effects	drowsiness, lightheadedness, confusion, *dependance,* after IV injection there may be a fall in blood pressure and severe respiratory depression

Interactions	*alcohol* – enhances sedative effect *anaesthesia* – enhances sedative effect *antiepileptics* – reported to both increase and decrease plasma phenytoin concentration *antihistamines* – enhanced sedative effect *antihypertensives* – enhanced hypotensive effect
Fetal risk	teratogen in the first and second trimesters, prolonged use in the third trimester may cause neonatal respiratory depression, drowsiness, hypotonia and withdrawal
Breastfeeding	avoid repeated doses and observe the infant for lethargy and weight loss

B.P.	phenytoin
Proprietary	EPANUTIN ®
Group	antiepileptic
Uses/indications	epilepsy, eclampsia
Type of drug	PoM
Presentation	capsules, tablets, suspension
Dosage	see local protocols
Route of admin.	oral, IV infusion or injection, p.r.
Contra-ind.	see chapter 6
Side effects	see chapter 6
Interactions	see chapter 6
Fetal risk	see chapter 6
Breastfeeding	see chapter 6

B.P.	chlorimethiazole
Proprietary	HEMINEVRIN ®
Group	hypnotic, anxiolytic
Uses/indications	eclampsia
Type of drug	PoM
Presentation	capsules, syrup, IV infusion
Dosage	see local protocol
Route of admin.	IV (oral)
Contra-ind.	pulmonary insufficiency
Side effects	
Interactions	*alcohol* – enhances the sedative effect *anaesthesia* – enhances the sedative effect *analgesics* – opioids enhance the sedative effect *antihistamines* – enhance the sedative effect *antihypertensives* – enhance the hypotensive effect
Fetal risk	can depress neonatal respiration
Breastfeeding	amount secreted too small to be harmful

Treatment of severe haemorrhage

B.P.	carboprost
Proprietary	HAEMABATE ®
Group	prostaglandin
Uses/indications	postpartum haemorrhage unresponsive to ergometrine or syntocinon
Type of drug	PoM
Presentation	ampoules
Dosage	250 micrograms repeated as required at 90 minute intervals – in severe loss not less than 15 minutes total dose is 2 mg maximum i.e. 8 doses
Route of admin.	IM
Contra-ind.	cardiac, pulmonary hepatic disease
Side effects bronchospasm	multiple including nausea, vomiting, hyperthermia, flushing,
Interactions	
Fetal risk	not applicable
Breastfeeding	not applicable

Drugs used in the treatment of cardiac arrest

These drugs can be split into three sections, those used in primary treatment of cardiac arrest, those administered as secondary to stabilize the patients condition, and those administered in the treatment of anaphylactic shock.

Primary

B.P.	adrenaline (epinephrine)
Proprietary	EPPY SIMPLENE ®
Group	
Uses/indications	asystolic cardiac arrest in conjunction with calcium chloride and defibrillation. It increases cardiac output and the force of contractility by producing generalized vasoconstriction by action on vascular smooth muscle. Can also be used in anaphylactic shock or severe allergic reactions.
Type of drug	
Presentation	Minijet or ampoules
Dosage	0.5–1 ml of 1:10 000
Route of admin.	IV
Contra-ind.	
Side effects	anxiety, tremor, increased heart rate, cold peripheries, increased blood pressure
Interactions	
Fetal risk	
Breastfeeding	

Primary

B.P.	lignocaine
Proprietary	XYLOCAINE ®
Group	
Uses/indications	after acute myocardial infarction it suppresses ventricular arrythmias and reduces the potential for fibrillation and its recurrence. It decreases myocardial contractility and arterial blood pressure and can be used where there is persistent ventricular fibrillation or ventricular tachycardia
Presentation	Minijet , ampoules
Dosage	slow over 2 minutes – 1 mg/kg – bolus 0.5 mg/kg after 5–10 minutes
Route of admin.	
Contra-ind.	
Side effects	
Interactions	
Fetal risk	
Breastfeeding	

Primary

B.P.	atropine sulphate
Proprietary	
Group	
Uses/indications	it increases the heart rate by blocking the action of the vagus nerve on the sinus node. It is used in sinus bradycardia especially where there is a drop in blood pressure following myocardial infarction. It can also be used in asystolic cardiac arrest which is unresponsive to DC shock
Type of drug	
Presentation	Minijet – injection
Dosage	1–3 mg
Route of admin.	
Contra-ind.	
Side effects	
Interactions	
Fetal risk	
Breastfeeding	

Primary/secondary

B.P.	calcium carbonate/calcium gluconate
Proprietary	
Group	
Uses/indications	the calcium ions help to increase myocardial contractility when adrenaline has failed. Can be used in conjunction with adrenaline and defibrillation
Type of drug	
Presentation	
Dosage	
Route of admin.	
Contra-ind.	
Side effects	
Interactions	
Fetal risk	
Breastfeeding	

Secondary

B.P.	bicarbonate – usually sodium
Proprietary	
Group	
Uses/indications	used to combat metabolic acidosis after cardiac arrest. Should not be given until 20 minutes of cardiac arrest has elapsed
Type of drug	
Presentation	
Dosage	
Route of admin.	
Contra-ind.	
Side effects	
Interactions	
Fetal risk	
Breastfeeding	

Anaphylaxis

B.P.	hydrocortisone
Proprietary	SOLU-CORTEF ®, HYDROCORTON ®, EFCORTESOL ®
Group	corticosteroids
Uses/indications	in anaphylaxis, in suppression of the inflammatory response
Type of drug	
Presentation	ampoules
Dosage	*IV* – 100–300 mg
Route of admin.	IM, IV
Contra-ind.	
Side effects	
Interactions	
Fetal risk	
Breastfeeding	

Anaphylaxis

B.P.	chlorpheniramine
Proprietary	PIRITON ®
Group	antihistamine – see chapter 12
Uses/indications	in anaphylaxis, in suppression of severe inflammatory response
Type of drug	
Presentation	see chapter 12
Dosage	continuous IV infusion over 24 hrs
Route of admin.	
Contra-ind.	
Side effects	
Interactions	
Fetal risk	
Breastfeeding	

Drugs used in neonatal resuscitation

B.P.	naloxone
Proprietary	NARCAN ®
Group	antagonist of central and respiratory depression
Uses/indications	reversal of the effects of opioid analgesia in neonates
Type of drug	PoM
Presentation	ampoules
Dosage	200 micrograms single dose at birth This dose is for a term infant only and a pre-term infant requires a smaller dose – this should be agreed with the paediatrician in attendance at delivery
Route of admin.	IM, sub cutaneous
Contra-ind.	
Side effects	
Interactions	
Fetal risk	
Breastfeeding	

References

Baskett, P.J.F. (1993). *Resuscitation Handbook.* 2nd Edition. London: Mosby-Wolfe.

Briggs, G.G., Freeman, R.K., Yaffe, S.J. (1990). *Drugs In Pregnancy And Lactation: A Reference Guide To Fetal And Neonatal Risk.* 3rd edition. Baltimore: Williams and Wilkins.

British Medical Association and the Royal Pharmaceutical Society of Great Britain (1996). *British National Formulary.* No. 31, March, Avon: Bath Press.

Hopkins, S.J. (1995). *Drugs And Pharmacology For Nurses.* 12th edition. Edinburgh: Churchill Livingstone.

Further reading

Chalmers, I., Grant, A. (1996). 'Salutory lessons from the collaborative eclampsia trial'. *Evidence Based Medicine,* Vol. 1, No. 2, Jan/Feb, pp. 39–40. *MIDIRS Midwifery Digest,* June, Vol. 6, No. 2, pp. 181–183.

Index

Syntocinon 101
  infusions 95
  overdose 100
Syntometrine 102
syphilis 37

T

Tagamet 7, 153
temazepam 134
terbutaline 113
terfenadine 86
Terfenor 86
Terfox 86
termination
  therapeutic 107
thromboembolism 40
thrush 142
thyroid hormone 147
thyroxine 147
Trandate 63
trichomonas vaginalis 38
tricyclic antidepressants 53
Triludan 86
Tylex 27

U

UKCC Guidelines for the
  Administration of Medicine
  (1992) 2
Unihep 41
urticaria 84, 85, 86
uterine cervix 105
uterine hyperstimulation 101
UTI 33

V

vaccination 122
vaccines 122
  immunoglobulin 124
  live 123
  rubella 123
vagus nerve 163

Valium 156
varicella 122
  zoster 149
  zoster immunoglobulin 124
varicosities 141
vasodilator 62
Velosef 36
Ventolin 112
  hydroxocobalamin 127
vitamins 126
  B12 126
    deficiency 127
  C 126, 129
  K 126
  B complex 127, 128
Voltarol 23
vomiting 56, 57

W

warfarin sodium 42
Warfarin wbp 42
water 95
  intoxication 101
withdrawal symptoms 19, 20

X

Xylocaine 12, 162

Y

Yutopar 110

Z

Zadstadt 38
Zantac 8
zidovudine (AZT) 150
Zovirax 149